EBOLA VIRUS DISEASE: FROM EPIDEMIC TO PANDEMIC

Thomas Jerome Baker

DEDICATION

This book is dedicated to every human being on the planet.

Its purpose is to inform people about Ebola Virus Disease (EVD). It seeks to give the best possible information about Ebola from a variety of perspectives. To do this, it relies heavily on authoritative sources.

It brings together health information, medical information, humanitarian concerns, social media and the economic impact of the Ebola epidemic.

Most importantly, it helps to raise international awareness that Africa needs help to get the disease under control. In the words of Physician Assistant Jackson Niamiah: "We cannot fight Ebola alone. You, the international community, must help us. If the international community does not stand up, we will be wiped out."

CONTENTS

ACKNOWLEDGMENTS

Addressing the Myths

"It can't be stopped!" False. Previous outbreaks have been stopped much sooner. Officials didn't realize that Ebola had broken out in West Africa.

"It's airborne!" False. It's not airborne. While you can get sick if someone sneezes or coughs right into your face, this is rare.

"Everyone who gets Ebola dies!" No, they don't. Dr. Kent Brantley survived. In fact, close to half of the people who come down with Ebola actually do survive. Getting immediate medical care is vital to survival.

"It's easy to get Ebola!" No. Again, read up on how Ebola is transmitted. People who get Ebola aren't contagious until they develop symptoms. Here's a quick comparison:

-- One person with measles could potentially infect 17 people.
-- People sick with Ebola infect one or two people on average.

I ask you one thing: The next time someone tries to get you panicked about Ebola, tell them the real facts. Calm down. (Source: "Is Ebola Scaring You?" by Barbara Alvarez) Click this link for full story: http://huff.to/1vZUk9q

1 SOMETHING NEVER SEEN BEFORE

In September 1976, a package containing a shiny, blue thermos flask arrived at the Institute of Tropical Medicine in Antwerp, Belgium. Working in the lab that day was Peter Piot, a 27-year-old scientist and medical school graduate who was training as a clinical microbiologist.

"It was just a normal flask like any other you would use to keep coffee warm," recalls Piot, now Director of the London School of Hygiene and Tropical Medicine.

But this thermos wasn't carrying coffee - inside was an altogether different cargo.

Nestled amongst a few melting ice cubes were vials of blood along with a note. It was from a Belgian doctor based in what was then Zaire, now the Democratic Republic of Congo - his handwritten message explained that the blood was that of a nun, also from Belgium, who had fallen ill with a mysterious illness which he couldn't identify.

This unusual delivery had travelled all the way from Zaire's capital city Kinshasa, on a commercial flight, in one of the passengers' hand luggage.

"When we opened the thermos, we saw that one of the vials was broken and blood was mixing with the water from the melted ice," says Piot.

He and his colleagues were unaware just how dangerous that was. As the blood leaked into the icy water so too did a deadly unknown virus. The samples were treated like numerous others the lab had tested before, but when the scientists placed some of the cells under an electron microscope they saw something they didn't expect.

"We saw a gigantic worm like structure - gigantic by viral standards," says Piot. "It's a very unusual shape for a virus, only one other virus looked like that and that was the Marburg virus."

The Marburg virus was first recognised in 1967 when 31 people became ill with haemorrhagic fever in the cities of Marburg and Frankfurt in Germany and in Belgrade, the capital of Yugoslavia. This Marburg outbreak was associated with laboratory staff who were working with infected monkeys imported from

Uganda - seven people died.

Piot knew how serious Marburg could be - but after consulting experts around the world he got confirmation that what he was seeing under the microscope wasn't Marburg - this was something else, something never seen before... (Source: BBC News) Click this link for full story => http://bbc.in/1sqeI2s

**

An epidemic of Ebola virus disease (EVD) is ongoing in certain West African countries. It began in Guinea in December 2013 then spread to Liberia and Sierra Leone.[4]Much smaller subsidiary outbreaks have occurred in Senegal and Nigeria, with individual cases in the United States and Spain.[3][5]

As of October 2014, the World Health Organization (WHO), the United States Centers for Disease Control and Prevention (CDC) and local governments reported a total of 8,399 suspected cases and 4,033 deaths (4,633 cases and 2,423 deaths having been laboratory confirmed),[2] though the WHO believes that this substantially understates the magnitude of the outbreak[6] with possibly 2.5 times as many cases as have been reported.[7]

The current epidemic of EVD, caused by Ebola virus, is the most severe outbreak of Ebola since the discovery of ebolaviruses in 1976,[8] and by September 2014 cases of EVD from this single outbreak exceeded the sum of all previously identified cases.[9] The epidemic has caused significant mortality, with a Case Fatality Rate (CFR) reported as 71%.[4]

Affected countries have encountered many difficulties in their control efforts. The WHO has estimated that region's capacity for treating EVD is insufficient by the equivalent of 2,122 beds.[10] In some areas, people have become suspicious of both the government and hospitals; some hospitals have been attacked by angry protestors who believe that the disease is a hoax or that the hospitals are responsible for the disease.

Many of the areas that are seriously affected with the outbreak are areas of extreme poverty with limited access to soap or running water to help control the spread of disease.[11] Other factors include belief in traditional folk remedies, and cultural practices that involve physical contact with the deceased, especially <u>death customs</u> such as <u>washing the body of the deceased</u>.[12][13][14] Some hospitals lack basic supplies and are understaffed. This has increased the chance of staff catching the virus themselves. In August, the WHO reported that ten percent of the dead have been health care workers.[15]

By the end of August, the WHO reported that the loss of so many health workers was making it difficult for them to provide sufficient numbers of foreign medical staff.[16]

By September 2014, <u>Médecins Sans Frontières</u>, the largest <u>NGO</u> working in the affected regions, had grown increasingly critical of the international response. Speaking on 3 September, the international president spoke out concerning the lack of assistance from the <u>United Nations</u> member countries saying, "Six months into the worst Ebola epidemic in history, the world is losing the battle to contain it."[17]

A United Nations spokesperson stated "they could stop the Ebola outbreak in West Africa in 6 to 9 months, but only if a 'massive' global response is implemented."[18]

The Director-General of the WHO, <u>Margaret Chan</u>, called the outbreak "the largest, most complex and most severe we've ever seen" and said that it "is racing ahead of control efforts".[18]

In a 26 September statement, the WHO said, "The Ebola epidemic ravaging parts of West Africa is the most severe acute public health emergency seen in modern times."[19]

Source: "Ebola Virus Epidemic in West Africa" Click this link for full story: => http://bit.ly/1qdm7NW

**

Ebola is scaring me. Why? I live in Chile, a country which I have grown accustomed to referring to as, "The End Of The World". I should be feeling relatively safe. Yet when news reports begin to increase their frequency of reporting on Ebola Virus Disease (EVD), I sit up and take notice. One idiosyncrasy of life in Chile is that there is always a Chilean who somehow gets involved in every major world event. So now would be the best time to prepare myself, before we have the first case of EVD in Chile, by informing myself thoroughly about EVD.

2 EBOLA VIRUS DISEASE

Key facts

Ebola virus disease (EVD), formerly known as Ebola haemorrhagic fever, is a severe, often fatal illness in humans.

The virus is transmitted to people from wild animals and spreads in the human population through human-to-human transmission.

The average EVD case fatality rate is around 50%. Case fatality rates have varied from 25% to 90% in past outbreaks.

The first EVD outbreaks occurred in remote villages in Central Africa, near tropical rainforests, but the most recent outbreak in west Africa has involved major urban as well as rural areas.

Community engagement is key to successfully controlling outbreaks. Good outbreak control relies on applying a package of interventions, namely case management, surveillance and contact tracing, a good laboratory service, safe burials and social mobilisation.

Early supportive care with rehydration, symptomatic treatment improves survival. There is as yet no licensed treatment proven to neutralise the virus but a range of blood, immunological and drug therapies are under development.

There are currently no licensed Ebola vaccines but 2 potential candidates are undergoing evaluation.

Background

The Ebola virus causes an acute, serious illness which is often fatal if untreated. Ebola virus disease (EVD) first appeared in 1976 in 2 simultaneous outbreaks, one in Nzara, Sudan, and the other in Yambuku, Democratic Republic of Congo. The latter occurred in a village near the Ebola River, from which the disease takes its name.

The current outbreak in West Africa, (first cases notified in March 2014), is the largest and most complex Ebola outbreak since the Ebola virus was first discovered in 1976. There have been more cases and deaths in this outbreak than all others combined. It has also spread between countries starting in Guinea then spreading across land borders to Sierra Leone and Liberia, by air (1 traveller only) to Nigeria, and by land (1 traveller) to Senegal.

The most severely affected countries, Guinea, Sierra Leone and Liberia have very weak health systems, lacking human and infrastructural resources, having only recently emerged from long periods of conflict and instability. On August 8, the WHO Director-General declared this outbreak a Public Health Emergency of International Concern.

A separate, unrelated Ebola outbreak began in Boende, Equateur, an isolated part of the Democratic Republic of Congo.

The virus family Filoviridae includes 3 genera: Cuevavirus, Marburgvirus, and Ebolavirus. There are 5 species that have been identified: Zaire, Bundibugyo, Sudan, Reston and Taï Forest. The first 3, Bundibugyo ebolavirus, Zaire ebolavirus, and Sudan ebolavirus have been associated with large outbreaks in Africa. The virus causing the 2014 west African outbreak belongs to the Zaire species.

Transmission

It is thought that fruit bats of the Pteropodidae family are natural Ebola virus hosts. Ebola is introduced into the human population through close contact with the blood, secretions, organs or other bodily fluids of infected animals such as chimpanzees, gorillas, fruit bats, monkeys, forest antelope and porcupines found ill or dead or in the rainforest.

Ebola then spreads through human-to-human transmission via direct contact (through broken skin or mucous membranes) with the blood, secretions, organs or other bodily fluids of infected people, and with surfaces and materials (e.g. bedding, clothing) contaminated with these fluids.

Health-care workers have frequently been infected while

treating patients with suspected or confirmed EVD. This has occurred through close contact with patients when infection control precautions are not strictly practiced.

Burial ceremonies in which mourners have direct contact with the body of the deceased person can also play a role in the transmission of Ebola.

People remain infectious as long as their blood and body fluids, including semen and breast milk, contain the virus. Men who have recovered from the disease can still transmit the virus through their semen for up to 7 weeks after recovery from illness.

Symptoms of Ebola virus disease

The incubation period, that is, the time interval from infection with the virus to onset of symptoms is 2 to 21 days.

Humans are not infectious until they develop symptoms. First symptoms are the sudden onset of fever fatigue, muscle pain, headache and sore throat. This is followed by vomiting, diarrhoea, rash, symptoms of impaired kidney and liver function, and in some cases, both internal and external bleeding (e.g. oozing from the gums, blood in the stools). Laboratory findings include low white blood cell and platelet counts and elevated liver enzymes.

Diagnosis

It can be difficult to distinguish EVD from other infectious diseases such as malaria, typhoid fever and meningitis. Confirmation that symptoms are caused by Ebola virus infection are made using the following investigations:

antibody-capture enzyme-linked immunosorbent assay (ELISA)
antigen-capture detection tests
serum neutralization test
reverse transcriptase polymerase chain reaction (RT-PCR) assay
electron microscopy
virus isolation by cell culture.

Samples from patients are an extreme biohazard risk; laboratory testing on non-inactivated samples should be conducted under maximum biological containment conditions.

Treatment and vaccines

Supportive care-rehydration with oral or intravenous fluids- and treatment of specific symptoms, improves survival. There is as yet no proven treatment available for EVD. However, a range of potential treatments including blood products, immune therapies and drug therapies are currently being evaluated. No licensed vaccines are available yet, but 2 potential vaccines are undergoing human safety testing.

Prevention and control

Good outbreak control relies on applying a package of interventions, namely case management, surveillance and contact tracing, a good laboratory service, safe burials and social mobilisation. Community engagement is key to successfully controlling outbreaks. Raising awareness of risk factors for Ebola infection and protective measures that individuals can take is an effective way to reduce human transmission. Risk reduction messaging should focus on several factors:

Reducing the risk of wildlife-to-human transmission from contact with infected fruit bats or monkeys/apes and the consumption of their raw meat. Animals should be handled with gloves and other appropriate protective clothing. Animal products (blood and meat) should be thoroughly cooked before consumption.

Reducing the risk of human-to-human transmission from direct or close contact with people with Ebola symptoms, particularly with their bodily fluids. Gloves and appropriate personal protective equipment should be worn when taking care of ill patients at home. Regular hand washing is required after visiting patients in hospital, as well as after taking care of patients at home.

Outbreak containment measures including prompt and safe

burial of the dead, identifying people who may have been in contact with someone infected with Ebola, monitoring the health of contacts for 21 days, the importance of separating the healthy from the sick to prevent further spread, the importance of good hygiene and maintaining a clean environment.

Controlling infection in health-care settings:

Health-care workers should always take standard precautions when caring for patients, regardless of their presumed diagnosis. These include basic hand hygiene, respiratory hygiene, use of personal protective equipment (to block splashes or other contact with infected materials), safe injection practices and safe burial practices.

Health-care workers caring for patients with suspected or confirmed Ebola virus should apply extra infection control measures to prevent contact with the patient's blood and body fluids and contaminated surfaces or materials such as clothing and bedding. When in close contact (within 1 metre) of patients with EBV, health-care workers should wear face protection (a face shield or a medical mask and goggles), a clean, non-sterile long-sleeved gown, and gloves (sterile gloves for some procedures).

Laboratory workers are also at risk. Samples taken from humans and animals for investigation of Ebola infection should be handled by trained staff and processed in suitably equipped laboratories.

WHO response

WHO aims to prevent Ebola outbreaks by maintaining surveillance for Ebola virus disease and supporting at-risk countries to developed preparedness plans. The document provides overall guidance for control of Ebola and Marburg virus outbreaks:

Ebola and Marburg virus disease epidemics: preparedness, alert, control, and evaluation

When an outbreak is detected WHO responds by supporting surveillance, community engagement, case management, laboratory services, contact tracing, infection control, logistical support and training and assistance with safe burial practices.

WHO has developed detailed advice on Ebola infection prevention and control:

Infection prevention and control guidance for care of patients with suspected or confirmed Filovirus haemorrhagic fever in health-care settings, with focus on Ebola

Overview

This document provides a summary of infection control recommendations when providing direct and non-direct care to patients with suspected or confirmed Filovirus haemorrhagic fever, including Ebola or Marburg haemorrhagic fevers. These recommendations are interim and will be updated when additional information becomes available. The sections of the guidance cover:

General patient care

Direct patient care (for suspected or confirmed patients with haemorrhagic fever)

Waste management

Non-patient care activities: diagnostic laboratory activities, movement and burial of human remains, post-mortem examinations, managing exposure to virus through body fluids, including blood.

Related links
http://bit.ly/1vhnGBp
All publications on Ebola
Ebola virus disease - website

3 QUESTIONS AND ANSWERS ON EBOLA

General

How do I protect myself against Ebola?

If you must travel to an area affected by the 2014 Ebola outbreak, protect yourself by doing the following:

Wash hands frequently or use an alcohol-based hand sanitizer.

Avoid contact with blood and body fluids of any person, particularly someone who is sick.

Do not handle items that may have come in contact with an infected person's blood or body fluids.

Do not touch the body of someone who has died from Ebola.

Do not touch bats and nonhuman primates or their blood and fluids and do not touch or eat raw meat prepared from these animals.

Avoid hospitals in West Africa where Ebola patients are being treated. The U.S. Embassy or consulate is often able to provide advice on medical facilities.

Seek medical care immediately if you develop fever (temperature of 101.5°F/ 38.6°C) and any of the other following symptoms: headache, muscle pain, diarrhea, vomiting, stomach pain, or unexplained bruising or bleeding.

Limit your contact with other people until and when you go to the doctor. Do not travel anywhere else besides a healthcare facility.

For general information about Ebola, please use the links below:

Ebola Virus Disease: From Epidemic to Pandemic

About Ebola
Signs and Symptoms
Transmission
Risk of Exposure
Prevention

CDC has issued a Warning, Level 3 travel notice for U.S. citizens to avoid nonessential travel to Guinea, Liberia, and Sierra Leone.

CDC has downgraded the travel notice for Nigeria to a Watch, Level 1 because of the decreased risk of Ebola in Nigeria. Travelers to Nigeria should practice usual precautions.

CDC has also issued an Alert, Level 2 travel notice for the Democratic Republic of the Congo (DRC). A small number of Ebola cases have been reported in the DRC, though current information indicates that this outbreak is not related to the ongoing Ebola outbreak in West Africa.

For travel notices and other information for travelers, visit the Travelers' Health Ebola web page.

Has the first patient to become sick in this outbreak, know as "patient zero" been identified?

Reports in the medical literature and elsewhere have attempted to identify the patient who might have been the initial person infected in the West Africa Ebola outbreak. It's important for CDC to learn as much as it can about the source and initial spread of any outbreak.

With regard to the West Africa Ebola outbreak, tracing the lineage of how Ebola has spread thus far can help CDC apply that knowledge toward better prevention and care techniques. The knowledge gained in this work might entail details about specific patients. CDC generally refrains, however, from identifying particular patients in any aspect of an outbreak.

What is CDC doing in the U.S. about the outbreak in West Africa?

CDC has activated its Emergency Operations Center (EOC) to help coordinate technical assistance and control activities with partners. CDC has deployed several teams of public health experts to the West Africa region and plans to send additional public health experts to the affected countries to expand current response activities.

If an ill traveler arrives in the U.S., CDC has protocols in place to protect against further spread of disease. These protocols include having airline crew notify CDC of ill travelers on a plane before arrival, evaluation of ill travelers, and isolation and transport to a medical facility if needed. CDC, along with Customs & Border Patrol, has also provided guidance to airlines for managing ill passengers and crew and for disinfecting aircraft. CDC has issued a Health Alert Notice reminding U.S. healthcare workers about the importance of taking steps to prevent the spread of this virus, how to test and isolate patients with suspected cases, and how to protect themselves from infection.

Infection Control

Can hospitals in the United States care for an Ebola patient?

Any U.S. hospital that is following CDC's infection control recommendations and can isolate a patient in their own room with a private bathroom is capable of safely managing a patient with Ebola.

Travelers

What is being done to prevent ill travelers in West Africa from getting on a plane?

In West Africa

CDC's Division of Global Migration and Quarantine (DGMQ) is working with airlines, airports, and ministries of health to provide technical assistance for the development of exit screening and travel restrictions in the affected areas. This includes:

Assessing the ability of Ebola-affected countries and airports to conduct exit screening,

Assisting with development of exit screening protocols,

Training staff on exit screening protocols and appropriate PPE use, and

Training in-country staff to provide future trainings.

During Travel

CDC works with international public health organizations, other federal agencies, and the travel industry to identify sick travelers arriving in the United States and take public health actions to prevent the spread of communicable diseases. Airlines are required to report any deaths onboard or ill travelers meeting certain criteria to CDC before arriving into the United States, and CDC and its partners determine whether any public health action is needed.

If a traveler is infectious or exhibiting symptoms during or after a flight, CDC will conduct an investigation of exposed travelers and work with the airline, federal partners, and state and local health departments to notify them and take any necessary public health action. When CDC receives a report of an ill traveler on a cruise or cargo ship, CDC officials work with the shipping line to make an assessment of public health risk and to coordinate any necessary response.

In the United States

CDC has staff working 24/7 at 20 Border Health field offices located in international airports and land borders. CDC staff are ready 24/7 to investigate cases of ill travelers on planes and ships

Thomas Jerome Baker

entering the United States.

CDC works with partners at all ports of entry into the United States to help prevent infectious diseases from being introduced and spread in the United States. CDC works with Customs and Border Protection, U.S. Department of Agriculture, U.S. Coast Guard, U.S. Fish and Wildlife Services, state and local health departments, and local Emergency Medical Services staff.

Relatively few of the approximately 350 million travelers who enter the United States each year come from these countries. Secondly, most people who become infected with Ebola are those who live with or care for people who have already caught the disease and are showing symptoms. CDC and healthcare providers in the United States are prepared for the remote possibility that a traveler could get Ebola and return to the U.S. while sick.

What do I do if I'm returning to the U.S. from the area where the outbreak is occurring?

After you return, pay attention to your health.

Monitor your health for 21 days if you were in an area with an Ebola outbreak, especially if you were in contact with blood or body fluids, items that have come in contact with blood or body fluids, animals or raw meat, or hospitals where Ebola patients are being treated or participated in burial rituals.

Seek medical care immediately if you develop fever (temperature of 101.5°F/ 38.6°C) and any of the following symptoms: headache, muscle pain, diarrhea, vomiting, stomach pain, or unexplained bruising or bleeding.

Tell your doctor about your recent travel and your symptoms before you go to the office or emergency room. Advance notice will help your doctor care for you and protect other people who may be in the office.

What do I do if I am traveling to an area where the

outbreak is occurring?

If you are traveling to an area where the Ebola outbreak is occurring, protect yourself by doing the following:

Wash your hands frequently or use an alcohol-based hand sanitizer.

Avoid contact with blood and body fluids of any person, particularly someone who is sick.

Do not handle items that may have come in contact with an infected person's blood or body fluids.

Do not touch the body of someone who has died from Ebola.

Do not touch bats and nonhuman primates or their blood and fluids and do not touch or eat raw meat prepared from these animals.

Avoid hospitals in West Africa where Ebola patients are being treated. The U.S. Embassy or consulate is often able to provide advice on facilities.

Seek medical care immediately if you develop fever (temperature of 101.5oF/ 38.6oC) and any of the other following symptoms: headache, muscle pain, diarrhea, vomiting, stomach pain, or unexplained bruising or bleeding.

Limit your contact with other people until and when you go to the doctor. Do not travel anywhere else besides a healthcare facility.

Should people traveling to Africa be worried about the outbreak?

Ebola has been reported in multiple countries in West Africa (see Affected Countries). CDC has issued a Warning, Level 3 travel notice for United States citizens to avoid all nonessential travel to Guinea, Liberia, and Sierra Leone.

A small number of cases were recently reported in Nigeria, but the virus does not appear to have been widely spread. CDC has downgraded the travel notice for Nigeria to a Watch, Level 1 because of the decreased risk of Ebola in Nigeria. Travelers to Nigeria should practice usual precautions.

CDC has also issued an Alert, Level 2 travel notice for the Democratic Republic of the Congo (DRC). A small number of Ebola cases have been reported in the DRC, though current information indicates that this outbreak is not related to the ongoing Ebola outbreak in West Africa. You can find more information on these travel notices at http://wwwnc.cdc.gov/travel/notices.

CDC currently does not recommend that travelers avoid visiting other African countries. Although spread to other countries is possible, CDC is working with the governments of affected countries to control the outbreak.

Ebola is a very low risk for most travelers – it is spread through direct contact with the blood or other body fluids of a sick person, so travelers can protect themselves by avoiding sick people and hospitals in West Africa where patients with Ebola are being treated.

Why were the ill Americans with Ebola brought to the U.S. for treatment? How is CDC protecting the American public?

A U.S. citizen has the right to return to the United States.

Although CDC can use several measures to prevent disease from being introduced in the United States, CDC must balance the public health risk to others with the rights of the individual. In this situation, the patients who came back to the United States for care were transported with appropriate infection control procedures in place to prevent the disease from being transmitted to others.

Ebola poses no substantial risk to the U.S. general population.

CDC recognizes that Ebola causes a lot of public worry and concern, but CDC's mission is to protect the health of all Americans, including those who may become ill while overseas. Ebola patients can be transported and managed safely when appropriate precautions are used.

What does CDC's Travel Alert Level 3 mean to U.S. travelers?

CDC recommends that U.S. residents avoid nonessential travel to Guinea, Liberia, and Sierra Leone. If you must travel (for example, to do for humanitarian aid work in response to the outbreak) protect yourself by following CDC's advice for avoiding contact with the blood and body fluids of people who are ill with Ebola. For more information about the travel alerts, see Travelers' Health Ebola web page.

Travel notices are designed to inform travelers and clinicians about current health issues related to specific destinations.

These issues may arise from disease outbreaks, special events or gatherings, natural disasters, or other conditions that may affect travelers' health. A level 3 alert means that there is a high risk to travelers and that CDC advises that travelers avoid nonessential travel.

In the United States

Are there any cases of people contracting Ebola in the U.S.?

CDC confirmed on September 30, 2014, the first travel-associated case of Ebola to be diagnosed in the United States. The person traveled from West Africa to Dallas, Texas, and later sought medical care at Texas Health Presbyterian Hospital of Dallas after developing symptoms consistent with Ebola. The medical facility has isolated the patient. Based on the person's travel history and symptoms, CDC recommended testing for Ebola.

CDC recognizes that even a single case of Ebola diagnosed in the United States raises concerns. Knowing the possibility exists, medical and public health professionals across the country have been preparing to respond. CDC and public health officials in Texas are taking precautions to identify people who have had close personal contact with the ill person and health care professionals have been reminded to use meticulous infection control at all times.

Is there a danger of Ebola spreading in the U.S.?

Ebola is not spread through casual contact; therefore, the risk of an outbreak in the U.S. is very low. We know how to stop Ebola's further spread: thorough case finding, isolation of ill people, contacting people exposed to the ill person, and further isolation of contacts if they develop symptoms.

The U.S. public health and medical systems have had prior experience with sporadic cases of diseases such as Ebola. In the past decade, the United States had 5 imported cases of Viral Hemorrhagic Fever (VHF) diseases similar to Ebola (1 Marburg, 4 Lassa). None resulted in any transmission in the United States.

Are people who were on the plane with this patient at risk?

A person must have symptoms to spread Ebola to others.

The ill person did not exhibit symptoms of Ebola during the flights from West Africa and CDC does not recommend that people on the same commercial airline flights undergo monitoring. The person reported developing symptoms five days after the return flight. CDC and public health officials in Texas are taking precautions to identify people who have had close personal contact with the ill person and health care professionals have been reminded to use meticulous infection control at all times.

Content source: Centers for Disease Control and Prevention

4 ECONOMIC IMPACT OF THE 2014 EBOLA EPIDEMIC: SHORT AND MEDIUM TERM ESTIMATES FOR WEST AFRICA

A report issued Wednesday by the World Bank forecasts that the total economic impact of Ebola could exceed $32 billion by the end of 2015 if the virus spreads from Liberia, Guinea and Sierra Leone to neighboring countries.

That single dollar amount doesn't fully convey the extraordinary human toll of a virus that kills four in five of its victims and could infect as many 1.4 million people by January. Yet the World Bank's estimate is a reminder that sickness and death are only part of what could be a developing regional crisis.

Already, farmers are abandoning their fields, and local authorities are restricting shipments of goods, according to the report. Fear of Ebola is spreading much faster than the virus itself, with what the report describes as potentially "catastrophic" economic consequences, including food shortages.

The World Bank's latest forecast elaborates on a previous report, adding new details and expanding the analysis to the region as a whole. The authors are optimistic that neighboring countries will be able to contain outbreaks, in which case the economic effects would be limited. They note that it is impossible to predict the spread of the virus and its effect on the economy with much confidence.

Source: The Washington Post
Click this link for full story: => http://wapo.st/1nhBRne

Executive Summary

Beyond the terrible toll in human lives and suffering, the Ebola epidemic currently afflicting West Africa is already having a measurable economic impact in terms of forgone output; higher fiscal deficits; rising prices; lower real household incomes and greater poverty. These economic impacts include the costs of healthcare and forgone productivity of those directly affected but, more importantly, they arise from the aversion behavior of others in response to the disease.

The **short-term (2014) impact** on output, estimated using on-the-ground data to inform revisions to sector-specific growth projections, is on the order of 2.1 percentage points (pp) of GDP in Guinea (reducing growth from 4.5 percent to 2.4 percent); 3.4 pp of GDP in Liberia (reducing growth from 5.9 percent to 2.5 percent) and 3.3 pp of GDP in Sierra Leone (reducing growth from 11.3 percent to 8.0 percent). This forgone output for these three countries corresponds to US$359 million in 2013 prices.

The short-term **fiscal impacts** are also large, at US$113 million (5.1 percent of GDP) for Liberia; US$95 million (2.1 percent of GDP for Sierra Leone) and US$120 million (1.8 percent of GDP) for Guinea. These estimates are best viewed as lower-bounds.

Slow containment scenarios would almost certainly lead to even greater impacts and corresponding financing gaps in both 2014 and 2015. Governments are mitigating some of these impacts on their budgets through reallocation of resources, but much international support is still needed.

As it is far from certain that the epidemic will be fully contained by December 2014 and in light of the considerable uncertainty about its future trajectory, two alternative scenarios are used to estimate the **medium-term (2015) impact** of the epidemic, extending to the end of calendar year 2015.

A "Low Ebola" scenario corresponds to rapid containment within the three most severely affected countries (henceforth the "core three countries"), while "High Ebola" corresponds to slower containment in the core three countries, with some broader regional contagion.

The medium-term impact (2015) on output in Guinea is estimated to be negligible under Low Ebola, and 2.3pp of GDP under High Ebola. In Liberia, it is estimated to be 4.2pp of GDP under Low Ebola, or 11.7pp of GDP under High Ebola.

In Sierra Leone, the impact would be 1.2pp of GDP under Low Ebola, and 8.9pp under High Ebola. The estimates of the GDP lost as a result of the epidemic in the core three countries (for calendar year 2015 alone) sum to US$97 million under Low Ebola (implying some recovery from 2014), and US$809 million under High Ebola (in 2013 dollars).

Over the medium term, however, both epidemiological and economic contagion in the broader sub-region of West Africa is likely. To account for the probable spillovers on neighboring countries, we use the Bank's integrated, multi-country general equilibrium model (LINKAGE), to estimate the **medium-term impact on output for West Africa as a whole.**

Under Low Ebola, the loss in GDP for the sub-region is estimated to be US$2.2 billion in 2014 and US$1.6 billion in 2015. Under High Ebola, the estimates are US$7.4 billion in 2014, and US$25.2 billion in 2015.

The take-away messages from this analysis are that the economic impacts are already very serious in the core three countries – particularly Liberia and Sierra Leone – and *could become catastrophic* under a slow-containment, High Ebola scenario.

In broader regional terms, the economic impacts could be limited if immediate national and international responses succeed in containing the epidemic and mitigating aversion behavior. The successful containment of the epidemic in Nigeria and Senegal so far is evidence that this is possible, given some existing health system capacity and a resolute policy response.

If, on the other hand, the epidemic spreads into neighboring countries, some of which have much larger economies, the cumulative two-year impact could reach US$32.6 billion by the end of 2015 – almost 2.5 times the combined 2013 GDP of the core three countries.

A swift policy reaction by the international community is crucial. With potential the economic costs of the Ebola epidemic being so high, very substantial containment and mitigation expenditures would be cost-effective, if they successfully avert the worst epidemiological outcomes.

To mitigate the medium term economic impact of the outbreak, current efforts by many partners to strengthen the health systems and fill the fiscal gaps in the core three countries are key priorities. These efforts should also be supplemented by investments in those countries and in their neighbors to renew the confidence of international tourism, travel, trade and investment partners.

Finally, there are two important caveats. First, this analysis does not take into account the longer term impacts generated by mortality, failure to treat other health conditions due to aversion behavior and lack of supply capacity, school closings and dropouts, and other shocks to livelihoods. It is truly focused on the short and medium-term inputs, over the next 18 months.

Second, these estimates are subject to considerable uncertainty, arising not only from the usual and well-known problems associated with economic forecasting and data scarcity, but also from the unusually high degree of uncertainty associated with the future epidemiological path of Ebola, and with people's behavioral responses to it.

All the analysis in this report therefore represents best-effort estimates under documented assumptions and modeling choices, but the margins of error associated with them are inevitably large. The scenarios should be read and interpreted accordingly.

(Source: The World Bank)
Cick this link for full report: => http://bit.ly/1vhzOT3

5 HOW YOU CAN AND CAN'T GET EBOLA

Here are the facts about how Ebola spreads, as outlined by the World Health Organisation (WHO), the US Centres for Disease Control and Prevention (CDC), and other official bodies.

You cannot get Ebola through the air

Ebola is not an airborne disease like influenza or chicken pox, and the WHO has categorically said reports suggesting that Ebola has mutated and become airborne are false.

"Airborne spread among humans implies inhalation of an infectious dose of virus from a suspended cloud of small dried droplets," it says.

"This mode of transmission has not been observed during extensive studies of the Ebola virus over several decades."

You cannot get Ebola through water
Ebola does not contaminate water supplies like cholera or dysentery do.

You cannot get Ebola from someone who is not already sick

The virus only appears in people's bodily fluids after they already have symptoms, so a carrier can't unknowingly spread it before they feel sick.

"The time from exposure to when signs or symptoms of the disease appear - the incubation period - is two to 21 days but the average time is eight to 10 days," the CDC says.

"Signs of Ebola include fever - higher than 38.6 degrees Celsius - and symptoms like severe headache, muscle pain, vomiting, diarrhea, stomach pain, or unexplained bleeding or bruising."

You cannot get Ebola from mosquitos

It isn't carried by insects the way dengue fever or Ross River fever are.

"There is no evidence that mosquitos or other insects can transmit Ebola virus," the CDC says. "Only mammals - for example, humans, bats, monkeys and apes - have shown the ability to spread and become infected with Ebola virus."

You cannot get Ebola from properly cooked food

Although Ebola has spread through the hunting, butchering and preparation of bush meat in Africa, it can't be transmitted through properly cooked food.

"If food products are properly prepared and cooked, humans cannot become infected by consuming them: the Ebola virus is inactivated through cooking," the WHO advises.

You can get Ebola from direct contact with the bodily fluids of an infectious person

This is the main method of transmission.

You can get Ebola if the blood, saliva, sweat, vomit, urine, semen or other bodily fluids of a sick person comes into direct contact with your broken skin or mucous membranes such as the mouth, nose, eyes or vagina.

Therefore, activities such as kissing, sharing food or having sex with an infectious person all provide potential for transmission. Needles are also a risk factor.

With Ebola, the most infectious bodily fluids are blood, faeces and vomit.

"The viral load in these fluids is enormous," notes Dominic Dwyer, the director of the Centre for Infectious Diseases in Sydney.

This means that healthcare workers who are treating Ebola patients, and the family and friends of infected people, are at the highest risk of getting sick.

If a person recovers from Ebola - the fatality rate in the current outbreak is about 50 per cent - sexual contact can remain risky.

"Men who have recovered from the disease can still transmit the virus through their semen for up to seven weeks after recovery from illness," the WHO says.

You can get Ebola from touching an infected surface

The Ebola virus can survive outside the body, so coming into direct contact with infected bodily fluids on surfaces such as bedding, clothing or furniture and then touching your eyes or mouth can spread the disease.

"Ebola is killed with hospital-grade disinfectants, such as household bleach," the CDC says.

"Ebola on dried on surfaces such as doorknobs and countertops can survive for several hours, however [the] virus in body fluids such as blood can survive up to several days at room temperature."

The virus can also survive on the skin of an infected person for several days, even after their death. The UK's National Health Service says this has meant traditional African burial rituals have played a part in Ebola's spread.

"The Ebola virus can survive for several days outside the body, including on the skin of an infected person, and it's common practice for mourners to touch the body of the deceased," the NHS says. "They only then need to touch their mouth to become infected."

You can (theoretically) get Ebola if an infectious person sneezes on you

"Common sense and observation tell us that spread of the virus via coughing or sneezing is rare, if it happens at all," the WHO says.

"Theoretically, wet and bigger droplets from a heavily infected individual, who has respiratory symptoms caused by other conditions or who vomits violently, could transmit the virus – over a short distance – to another nearby person.

"This could happen when virus-laden heavy droplets are directly propelled, by coughing or sneezing (which does not mean airborne transmission) onto the mucus membranes or skin with cuts or abrasions of another person.

"WHO is not aware of any studies that actually document this mode of transmission. On the contrary, good quality studies from previous Ebola outbreaks show that all cases were infected by direct close contact with symptomatic patients."

You can get Ebola from infected wild animals

In Africa, Ebola has spread to humans who eat infected wild animals without properly cooking them, or who otherwise come into contact with the bodily fluids of infected wild animals.

"It is thought that fruit bats of the Pteropodidae family are natural Ebola virus hosts," the WHO says.

"Ebola is introduced into the human population through close contact with the blood, secretions, organs or other bodily fluids of infected animals such as chimpanzees, gorillas, fruit bats, monkeys, forest antelope and porcupines found ill or dead or in the rainforest."

Also: viruses don't typically just 'go airborne'
Speculation that Ebola virus disease might mutate into a form that could easily spread among humans through the air is just that: speculation, unsubstantiated by any evidence.

World Health Organisation

In case you missed it, it bears repeating that Ebola is not an airborne disease.

The WHO also says viruses are not known for suddenly "becoming airborne", as some reports suggest Ebola has done.

"Scientists are unaware of any virus that has dramatically changed its mode of transmission," the WHO says.

"For example, the H5N1 avian influenza virus, which has caused sporadic human cases since 1997, is now endemic in chickens and ducks in large parts of Asia.

"That virus has probably circulated through many billions of birds for at least two decades. Its mode of transmission remains basically unchanged.

"Speculation that Ebola virus disease might mutate into a form that could easily spread among humans through the air is just that: speculation, unsubstantiated by any evidence."

Dr Dwyer from Sydney's Centre for Infectious Diseases says the pace of the current Ebola outbreak is in itself evidence that the disease is not airborne.

"The 'slowness' of spread in the current Ebola outbreak is against respiratory transmission being a major factor: the 2009 pandemic influenza virus, spread by respiratory droplets, had become worldwide in a comparable timeframe," he explains.

Numerous reports and social media posts have cited a 2012 study that found Ebola spread from pigs to monkeys without any direct contact as evidence the virus has "gone airborne".

However, the Canadian scientists behind that study themselves said the form of transmission they observed was not similar to influenza or other infections.

"If it was really an airborne virus like influenza is it would spread all over the place, and that's not happening," Dr Gary Kobinger from the Public Health Agency in Canada told the BBC in 2012.

"What we suspect is happening is large droplets - they can stay in the air, but not long, they don't go far," he explained.

"But they can be absorbed in the airway and this is how the infection starts, and this is what we think, because we saw a lot of evidence in the lungs of the non-human primates that the virus got in that way."

Oh, and Ebola zombies aren't real either

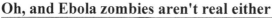

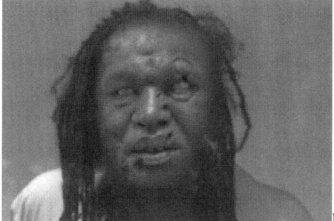

PHOTO: This image, said to be a man who came back to life after dying from Ebola, has gone viral. The story is not true.

In recent days, reports that three people who died from Ebola later rose from the dead have spread widely across social media: one report alone has been shared more than 500,000 times on Twitter and Facebook. It really should go without saying, but it is not real.

Snopes, the Independent, the Huffington Post and many, many others have the full debunking.

6 STOPPING EBOLA BEFORE IT TURNS INTO A PANDEMIC

Public-health workers will contain the Ebola case—and any secondary spread—diagnosed in Dallas. But the decisive risk to the U.S. will emerge in a few months. If the virus continues to spread in West Africa at its current pace, much larger global outbreaks will become likely.

Should these outbreaks coincide with the cold-weather peak of the flu season—when symptoms of influenza can be confused for the early signs of Ebola—the health-care system's ability to quarantine all the people with suspected Ebola infections, and test them in the required specially equipped labs, could be overwhelmed.

And if Ebola does decisively break out of West Africa, we may be unable to control the spread of the disease solely by conventional public-health tools of infection controls, tracking and tracing sick contacts, and isolating the ill. If this happens, we may face a global pandemic early next year.

The good news is that there are a number of promising therapeutics that have already shown activity against Ebola, from an immune-based drug called ZMapp that was given to seven infected patients, to at least two vaccines that appear ready for large-scale testing. ZMapp showed remarkable efficacy in bolstering the immune system to directly attack the virus in monkey experiments and may also have helped several Ebola sufferers recover.

Countries also need to agree on the standards for sanctioning an Ebola treatment. Here the WHO's policy-making apparatus may play a useful role in convening nations. Since the products will be first used on a wide scale in West Africa, health leaders from those nations need to play a prominent role in reaching a decision on the standards. But history suggests they will also look to Western regulatory experts for guidance.

One standard might turn on whether a product has shown that it can be safely administered and is active at reducing the progression or transmission of the virus. This is different than the FDA's "safe and effective" standard. Evidence of effectiveness that meets conventional standards may be unobtainable given the urgency, as well as the complexity, of running Ebola trials. Instead of the typical double-blind trial, patients treated with the newly certified therapeutics should be closely followed so we can see how well the products are working in the intermediate and longer term.

Finally, even while we focus on developing an Ebola remedy, we need to decide how it would be shared. Who would pay for the purchase of a successful drug or vaccine and who would assume liability for adverse events? Would international organizations buy the product at full price and then make it freely available? If so, would the U.S. or other contributing nations reserve doses for their citizens? Or would we send Africa all we have?

The U.S. has a national-security interest to treat the disease in Africa before it comes to America's shores. On the other hand, the American people would not likely tolerate having an insufficient supply if there was an outbreak at home. None of these difficult questions are being addressed. They must be.

The world's poor response to Ebola in West Africa, its reliance on faulty estimates and false confidence, has turned an outbreak into an epidemic and made a pandemic possible. Public-health officials say a drug or vaccine is elusive, and won't arrive in time to solve this crisis. They can't know this to be true—and the crisis could be a lot worse than they are predicting. A crash effort to develop a therapeutic may be all the U.S.—and the world—has to bet on.

Source: Wall Street Journal (Gottlieb and Troy)
Click this link for full story: => http://on.wsj.com/1nhDK3n

**

7 EBOLA: MASSIVE DEPLOYMENT NEEDED TO FIGHT EPIDEMIC IN WEST AFRICA

Bringing the spreading Ebola epidemic under control in West Africa will require a massive deployment of resources by regional governments and aid agencies, the international medical humanitarian organization Doctors Without Borders/Médecins Sans Frontières (MSF) said today, warning that it has reached the limit of what it can do to fight the deadly outbreak.

Ebola patients have been identified in more than 60 locations in Guinea, Sierra Leone, and Liberia, complicating efforts to treat patients and curb the outbreak. MSF is the only aid organization treating people affected by the virus, which can kill up to 90 percent of those infected.

"The epidemic is out of control," said Dr. Bart Janssens, MSF director of operations. "With the appearance of new sites in Guinea, Sierra Leone, and Liberia, there is a real risk of it spreading to other areas."

Since the outbreak began in March, MSF has treated 470 patients—215 of them confirmed cases—in specialized treatment centers.

However, MSF is having difficulty responding to the large number of new cases emerging in different locations.

"We have reached our limits," said Janssens. "Despite the human resources and equipment deployed by MSF in the three affected countries, we are no longer able to send teams to the new outbreak sites."

The scale of the current Ebola epidemic is unprecedented in terms of geographical distribution and the numbers of cases and deaths. There have been 528 cases and 337 deaths since the epidemic began, according to the latest World Health Organization (WHO) figures.

This is the first time that Ebola has broken out in the region. Local communities are still very frightened of the disease, viewing health facilities with suspicion. Meanwhile, a lack of understanding about how the disease spreads has resulted in people attending funerals where infection-control measures are not implemented.

Despite the presence of a number of organizations working to raise awareness about the disease, their activities have not yet managed to reduce public anxiety about Ebola.

Meanwhile, civil society and political and religious authorities are failing to acknowledge the scale of the epidemic, with few prominent figures spreading messages promoting the fight against the disease.

"The WHO, the affected countries, and neighboring countries must deploy the resources necessary for an epidemic of this scale," said Janssen. "In particular, qualified medical staff need to be made available, training in how to treat Ebola needs to be organized, and awareness-raising activities among the population need to be stepped up. Ebola is no longer a public health issue limited to Guinea. It is affecting the whole of West Africa."

In Guinea, MSF is supporting the health authorities by treating patients in Conakry, Télimélé, and Guéckédou. Additional treatment units have been built in Macenta, Kissidougou, and Dabola. MSF teams are responding to alerts in villages, raising awareness in communities, and offering psychological support to patients and their families. MSF is also supporting epidemiological surveillance.

In Sierra Leone, MSF is working with the Ministry of Health in constructing a 50-bed Ebola treatment center in Kailahun, due to open this week. Small transit care units have already been set up in Koidu and Daru, with a third to open soon in Buedu. MSF has also provided the Ministry of Health with supplies for the construction of additional treatment centers.

In Liberia, an MSF team has set up a treatment unit in Foya, in the north of the country, and another in JFK Hospital in Monrovia. MSF has also organized training courses and donated equipment.

MSF currently has some 300 international and national staff working in Guinea, Sierra Leone, and Liberia. It has sent more than 40 tons of equipment and supplies to the region to help fight the epidemic.

Source: Press Release (Doctors Without Borders, June 2014)
Click this link for full story: => http://bit.ly/ZzINRZ
Video: PBS NewsHour=> http://bit.ly/1vXLXcy

8 EBOLA: MSF PRESENTATION TO UN SECURITY COUNCIL

Speaking from Monrovia via live video link, Liberian Doctors Without Borders/Médecins Sans Frontières (MSF) physician's assistant Jackson Niamah addresses the UN Security Council during an emergency session on the Ebola crisis in West Africa.

I wish to thank Ambassador Power for inviting my organization, Médecins Sans Frontières, to address this gathering of nations who can help my people, my country, and my region.

I am honored to represent MSF. We welcome President Obama's Ebola response plan and hope for its immediate implementation. We also call upon all member states of the United Nations to similarly mobilize their capacities. With every day that passes, the epidemic spreads and destroys more lives.

I first heard about cases of Ebola in March. Soon after, the disease came here to Monrovia. From then on, people began dying.

My niece, Francila Kollie, and my cousin, Jounpu Lowea, both nurses, became infected at work. While they were able to receive treatment, they died in late July. So many of my close friends, university classmates, and colleagues have also died in recent months.

Since I have a medical background, I felt it was my responsibility to help my country. I am a team leader in MSF's treatment center in Monrovia. I have worked in the triage, assessing patients prior to admission, in the suspected cases tent, and with patients confirmed to have Ebola. Because there is no cure, we provide supportive care to patients, in the form of food, hydration, and basic treatment of symptoms. If treated early enough, their chances of survival are much better.

I cannot stand aside and watch my people die. But I, along with my colleagues here, cannot fight Ebola alone. You, the international community, must help us. I wish to illustrate the battle we face.

We have seen so many patients die. And they die alone, terrified, and without their loved ones at their side. As a medic, one must have a different way of coping. When I go inside the treatment center, I keep my focus on what the patients need. We try to attend first to those who are weaker, those who need more help to eat and drink, or those who need to speak to one of our counselors because they are so traumatized and frightened.

We are trying to treat as many people as we can, but there are not nearly enough treatment centers and patient beds. We have to turn people away. And they are dying at our front door.

Right now, as I speak, people are sitting at the gates of our centers, literally begging for their lives. They rightly feel alone, neglected, denied –left to die a horrible, undignified death.

We are failing the sick because there is not enough help on the ground. And we are failing those who will inevitably become infected, because we cannot care properly for the sick in safe, protected environments and prevent the spread of the virus.

One day this week, I sat outside the treatment center eating my lunch. I saw a boy approach the gate. A week ago his father died from Ebola. I could see that his mouth was red with blood. We had no space for him. When he turned away to walk into town, I thought to myself that this boy is going to take a taxi, and he is going to go home to his family, and he will infect them.

On my night shift this week, I saw a patient who had driven for around 12 hours in an ambulance because there was no other treatment center.

We urgently need to get the disease under control, and we need your help.

We need what is referred to as contact tracing, to follow up every person who has been in contact with someone who is sick with Ebola or has died from the virus. We need to raise awareness about this disease, because there has been so much denial, even now, and despite the international attention.

We need more care centers, so that everyone can find a bed and not have to stay at home and risk infecting their families. We need to get our medical staff trained in proper procedures so they can keep the centers running. We also need to get health services running, and to make sure that it is safe for health staff to go to work. We have seen too many health workers and ambulance drivers come into our centers as patients, facing the same fate.

So please send your helicopters, your centers, your beds, and your expert personnel. But know that we also need the basics. There are still homes in Monrovia that do not have soap, water, and buckets. Even these simple things could help curb the spread of the virus.

Ebola has affected every aspect of our lives. Schools and universities have shut down, along with civil services. I feel that the future of my country is hanging in the balance.

My wife works at JFK Hospital here in Monrovia. We are educating our children to protect themselves so that they will survive. As children of health workers, they can be an example to their peers.

I also ask you to be an example to your peers, as nations with the resources, assets, and skills required to stop this catastrophe.
We do not have the capacity to respond to this crisis on its own. If the international community does not stand up, we will be wiped out. We need your help. We need it now. Thank you.

Source: (Doctors Without Borders, September 2014)
Click this link for video: => http://bit.ly/1xEAHmE

9 CHECKLIST FOR PATIENTS BEING EVALUATED FOR EVD

Upon arrival to clinical setting/triage

Does patient have fever (subjective or ≥101.5°F)?

Does patient have compatible EVD symptoms such as headache, weakness, muscle pain, vomiting, diarrhea, abdominal pain or hemorrhage?

Has the patient traveled to an Ebola-affected area in the 21 days before illness onset?

Upon initial assessment

Isolate patient in single room with a private bathroom and with the door to hallway closed

Implement standard, contact, & droplet precautions

Notify the hospital Infection Control Program at _____

Report to the health department at _____

Conduct a risk assessment for: High-risk exposures

Percutaneous (e.g., needle stick) or mucous membrane exposure to blood or body fluids from an EVD patient

Direct skin contact with skin, blood or body fluids from an EVD patient

Processing blood or body fluids from an EVD patient without appropriate PPE

Direct contact with a dead body in an Ebola-affected area without appropriate PPE

Low-risk exposures

Household members of an EVD patient or others who had brief direct contact (e.g., shaking hands) with an EVD patient without appropriate PPE

Healthcare personnel in facilities with EVD patients who have been in care areas of EVD patients without recommended PPE

Use of personal protective equipment (PPE)

Use a buddy system to ensure that PPE is put on and removed safely

Before entering patient room, wear:

Gown (fluid resistant or impermeable)
Facemask
Eye protection (goggles or face shield)
Gloves

If likely to be exposed to blood or body fluids, additional PPE may include but isn't limited to:

Double gloving
Disposable shoe covers
Leg coverings

Upon exiting patient room

PPE should be carefully removed without contaminating one's eyes, mucous membranes, or clothing with potentially infectious materials
Discard disposable PPE
Re-useable PPE should be cleaned and disinfected per the manufacturer's reprocessing instructions
Hand hygiene should be performed immediately after removal of PPE

During aerosol-generating procedures

Limit number of personnel present
Conduct in an airborne infection isolation room
Don PPE as described above except use a NIOSH certified fit-tested N95 filtering facepiece respirator for respiratory protection or alternative (e.g., PAPR) instead of a facemask

Patient placement and care considerations

Maintain log of all persons entering patient's room
Use dedicated disposable medical equipment (if possible)
Limit the use of needles and other sharps
Limit phlebotomy and laboratory testing to those procedures essential for diagnostics and medical care
Carefully dispose of all needles and sharps in puncture-proof sealed containers
Avoid aerosol-generating procedures if possible
Wear PPE (detailed in center box) during environmental cleaning and use an EPA-registered hospital disinfectant with a label claim for non-enveloped viruses*

Initial patient management

Consult with health department about diagnostic EVD RT-PCR testing**

Consider, test for, and treat (when appropriate) other possible infectious causes of symptoms (e.g., malaria, bacterial infections)
Provide aggressive supportive care including aggressive IV fluid resuscitation if warranted
Assess for electrolyte abnormalities and replete
Evaluate for evidence of bleeding and assess hematologic and coagulation parameters
Symptomatic management of fever, nausea, vomiting, diarrhea, and abdominal pain
Consult health department regarding other treatment options

This checklist is not intended to be comprehensive.
Additions and modifications to fit local practice are encouraged.

Source: CDC
http://www.cdc.gov/vhf/ebola/pdf/checklist-patients-evaluated-us-evd.pdf

10 HOW WE CAN STOP EBOLA

Ban Ki-moon
Secretary General of the United Nations
October 23, 2014 http://linkd.in/1pfxMkO

The Ebola outbreak in Guinea, Liberia and Sierra Leone is the largest the world has ever seen, and transmission is rising exponentially. Since the start of the outbreak, the disease has infected almost 10,000 people and killed nearly 4,900. The disease has taken a severe toll on healthcare workers, with more than 400 infected and over 200 dead, and already fragile health systems are suffering. More people are dying from common, treatable medical conditions than from Ebola. The virus is also having a grave impact on economic progress and stability, with inflation and food prices rising.

From doctors and grave diggers to nurses and ambulance drivers, I salute the courage of the many medical and support personnel who are working at great personal risk on the front-lines of the Ebola epidemic. Day after day they step forward to care for the sick and help prevent the virus from spreading. We owe them an enormous debt of gratitude.

The UN stands with the people affected by Ebola – those who are infected, those who are caring for the sick, those who have lost loved ones and the people of Guinea, Liberia and Sierra Leone who are living under the constant fear of infection.

They have asked for urgent help and the international community is answering the call with a totally unprecedented response. The first-ever UN emergency health mission, known as UNMEER, is working to respond to immediate needs and coordinate action on the ground. Many countries have made major financial contributions; others have sent trained and experienced medical personnel to give support on the ground.

We have five priorities for an effective Ebola response -- stop the outbreak, treat the infected, ensure essential services, preserve stability and prevent outbreaks in non-affected countries.

To do all of this, we need a massive surge in assistance – in the form of mobile laboratories, vehicles, helicopters, protective equipment, trained medical personnel, medevac capacities and more.

I have launched an appeal for $1 billion, which is now 40 per cent funded. As a complementary measure, I have established a flexible, accountable, strategic and transparent trust fund for governments, businesses and foundations to channel their contributions. Commitments are coming in – some $49.5 million, but we need considerably more to finance critical unfunded priorities and help reduce the rate of Ebola transmission.

The private sector has an important role to play. The Business Engagement Guideoutlines the ways that businesses can contribute to efforts – financially, with in-kind donations, by directly providing assets or services and more.

Spreading even faster than Ebola is fear and misunderstanding. We need to raise awareness of the facts of Ebola and what can be done to stop it.

Many people are unsure about how Ebola is spread and whether it's safe to travel. The World Health Organization (WHO) is providing the answers to these questions and more. Follow them on Twitter and Facebook for regular updates.

Some also have questions about travel restrictions to and from Ebola-affected areas. Experience has shown that blanket travel bans don't work and can in fact impede our ability to contain the disease. The only way to end this crisis is to end the Ebola epidemic at its source – and that means stepping up and providing the assistance so badly needed in West Africa. Isolation only hampers international efforts to reach people in need.

This week, WHO officially declared Nigeria and Senegal free

of Ebola virus transmission, after 42 days without a single case. These success stories show that Ebola can be contained.

If you want to help, there are several ways that we as individuals -- and as global citizens -- can step up. Stay informed. Share the facts. If you can, make a donation to help the Ebola response. Qualified health workers can also volunteer to be part of the Ebola response on the ground in West Africa.

Every contribution and every show of support matters.

Find out more about the global Ebola crisis response. **Get information from the** World Health Organization. **Follow the United Nations on:** **LinkedIn** | **Twitter** | **Facebook** | **Google+** | **YouTube** | **Tumblr** | **Pinterest** |**Instagram**

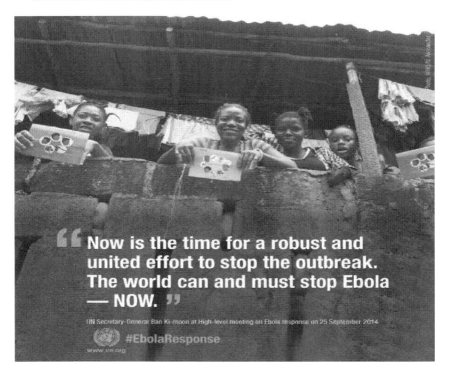

11
DR. STELLA AMEYO ADADEVOH: NIGERIA IS FREE OF EBOLA

This post first appeared on The Accra Report
By Accra Report Staff @accrareport
September 14, 2014

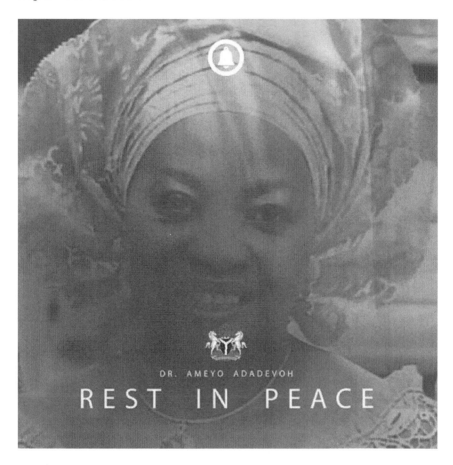

A requiem mass was held at the Christ the King Church on Friday, September 12, 2014 for Dr Ameyo Stella Adadevoh, the lead consultant physician and endocrinologist at the First Consultants Medical Centre in Lagos, Nigeria.

Dr Adadevoh contracted the Ebola Virus Disease (EVD) and died after coming into contact with a victim from Liberia.

The physician, who died on August 19, 2014, prevented Mr Patrick Sawyer, an American-Liberian who had arrived in Lagos en route to an ECOWAS meeting in Calabar, from leaving the medical centre when he showed symptoms of the EVD.

Her action was based on the fact that Mr Sawyer, who later died of the disease, posed a danger to members of the Nigerian public and the participants at the ECOWAS meeting.

She quarantined and treated Sawyer but unfortunately she contracted the disease which led to her death. She has since been buried in Nigeria.

A cousin of the late Dr Adadevoh, Mrs Sedina Tay-Agbozo, described her as a warm and friendly person who pursued any cause she believed in.

"She was committed and firm" she told the Daily Graphic and added that "By refusing to allow Mr Sawyer to leave the hospital, she prevented the disease from spreading."

An uncle of the late Dr Adadevoh and an Obstetrician Gynaecologist, Prof. Sydney Kobla Adadevoh, told the Daily Graphic that: "She put herself at risk and became a victim of the disease she was trying to prevent from spreading. She served for more than three decades, doing what she loved best—serving humanity."

Prof. Adadevoh said by identifying Mr Sawyer as a victim of the EVD in August, this year, Ameyo prevented a national catastrophe. She left a permanent mark on society and made solid her legacy as a courageous and patriotic heroine.

Brief biography

The late Dr Ameyo Stella Adadevoh was born on October 27,

1956 in Lagos, Nigeria. She was the first of four children.

Her paternal grandfather, an Anlo from Anyako and a staff of the United Africa Company (UAC), was transferred from the Gold Coast to Lagos in the early 1940s where he married the daughter of Herbert Macaulay, Nigerian nationalist.

The union produced many children including Prof. Babatunde Kwaku Adadevoh, a renowned Harvard University-trained physician and a former Vice Chancellor of the University of Lagos, who is Ameyo's father.

Ameyo's mother, Deborah Regina Mcintosh, is a niece of Nigeria's first President, Dr Nnamdi Azikiwe.

She was awarded a Bachelor of Medicine and Bachelor of Surgery degree by the University of Lagos in 1980.

In 1993, she completed a fellowship course in Endocrinology at Hammersmith Hospital of the Imperial College in London, UK.

For more than three decades, she practised as a medical doctor and for 21 of those years, she was the lead consultant physician and endocrinologist at the First Consultants Medical Centre in Obadele, Lagos.

Events leading to her death

Mr Sawyer was sent to the First Consultants Medical Centre in Lagos when he collapsed a few minutes after arriving in Lagos on his way to Calabar for an ECOWAS meeting.

The first impression that Dr Adadevoh had was that Mr Sawyer was suffering from malaria but other symptoms showed that he was not. She had an HIV test conducted on Mr Sawyer, which proved negative.

She then consulted senior medical practitioners who urged her to test for Ebola. The test proved positive.

Immense pressure was brought on Dr Adadevoh by the Liberian government to release Mr Sawyer to attend the meeting but she refused because he posed a danger to the public and had him isolated and later quarantined.

Tests conducted on Dr Adadevoh later proved that she had contracted the disease. She later fell into a coma and despite attempts to save her, she could not survive the scourge of the disease. She was an aunty to Radio Ghana's presidential correspondent Pascaline Ameyo Adadevoh.

May her soul rest in perfect peace…

**

Nigeria Is Free of Ebola

By Nick Cumming-Bruce
Oct. 20, 2014 http://nyti.ms/1xMDrhg

GENEVA — The World Health Organization declared Nigeria, Africa's most populous nation, officially free of Ebola infections on Monday, calling the outcome the triumphal result of "world-class epidemiological detective work."

The announcement came 42 days after the last reported infection in Nigeria's outbreak, twice the maximum incubation period for the Ebola virus.

The Nigerian response was upheld by the W.H.O. as an example of the measures other countries can take to halt the spread of the epidemic, which is concentrated in three West African countries: Guinea, Liberia and Sierra Leone.

"This is a spectacular success story that shows that Ebola can be contained," the W.H.O. said in a report on its website. But it also expressed caution that Nigeria cannot relax its defenses against the deadly virus.

12
IS EBOLA GOING TO KILL YOU?

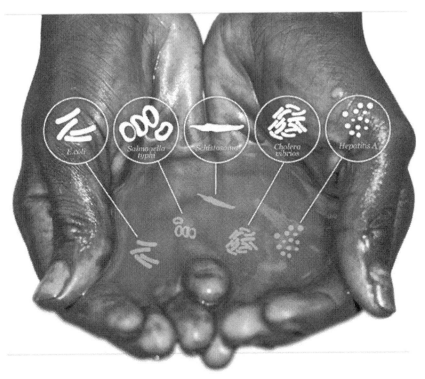

CAPE TOWN, South Africa – Ebola has grabbed all the headlines, but HIV still remains the world's deadliest infectious disease – **killing nearly the same number of people every day** that the Ebola outbreak in West Africa *has so far killed in 9 months…* http://bit.ly/1rLkxmr
First posted at The Richest
by Elyssa Rosadiuk Jan 3, 2014

Top 10 Leading Causes Of Death In 2013
Throughout history, various diseases, influenzas, and wars have plagued the world. The Black Plague decimated 14th century Europe with an estimated 75 million deaths. Small Pox, along with gunfire, wiped out an entire North American ethnic group. The Spanish Influenza claimed about 50 million lives around the world between the years of 1918-1920. About 50 million people, both

military and civilian alike, were killed in World War II. And even though Tuberculosis is no longer in the top 10 causes of death around the world, it was still the main cause behind the deaths of 1.3 million people in 2012.

Although the world has suffered through many fatalities, there are 10 leading causes of death that plague the world in a whole new way. They don't attack in waves, aren't really caused by just touching other people, and cause many to lose their loved ones. The order of the top 10 causes of death in a country, vary according to the country and the income class that you are researching, but around the world these are the top 10 leading causes of death for about 55% of the world's population.

10. Prematurity: 1.2 Million Deaths

Prematurity has claimed the title of 10th top causes of death around the world and is the leading cause behind 1.2 million deaths. If a child is born before 35 weeks, it is considered premature and the baby is usually kept in the hospital's intensive care unit. If a woman goes into labor before 37 weeks it is called preterm labor, and "late preterm" babies are born between 34-37 weeks, they are still handled carefully. Babies that do not look premature and are not put into intensive care, are still at risk for more problems than the full-term babies. Premature babies tend to have trouble breathing, feeding, and are more at risk of catching an infection.

If the mother has certain health conditions, such as diabetes, heart disease, and kidney disease, these may contribute to preterm labor. 15% of all premature births are multiple pregnancies (twins, triplets, etc.). Other factors that contribute to preterm labor include: a weakened cervix, birth defects in the uterus, history of preterm labor, infections (urinary tract, amniotic membrane, etc.), poor nutrition during pregnancy, high blood pressure, age (girls under 16, and woman older than 35), smoking, taking drugs, and being underweight all contribute to premature births.

November 17th is **World Prematurity Day** where countries raise awareness for prenatal care, and to honor preterm babies and their families. An average of 15 million babies were born prematurely in 2013, with an 8% of those infants dying. March of Dimes is the leading American organization in raising awareness for premature births.

9. Road Injury: 1.3 Million Deaths

Road injury is the leading cause of death for 1.3 million people. Road traffic accidents are the leading cause of death for young people between the ages of 15-29 years. About 91% of the world's road fatalities occur in low-income and middle-income countries, even though these countries only have about half of the world's vehicles. Approximately half of road related deaths are "vulnerable road users": pedestrians, cyclists, and motorcyclists. Only 28 countries (7% of the world's population), have adequate laws that address all 5 risk factors of road/vehicle deaths: speed, drunk-driving, helmets, seat belts, child restraints.

Distracted driving has also become a huge issue when it comes to road related injuries. It has in fact become the leading cause behind road related deaths. In the first 7 weeks of 2012, 9 people died on the road in Canada because of distractions such as texting while driving.

Russia, China, and India have the highest road related injury and deaths around the world. This has become such a big issue in Russia, cars actually have a Dash-Cam in order to tell whose fault an accident was.

8. HIV/AIDS: 1.63 Million Deaths

35.6 million people are living in the world with HIV, with an estimated 2.3 million newly affected. On top of that 1.63 million died from AIDS-related illnesses. 33% reduction since 2001 of newly affected people with HIV, while AIDS continues to severely impact countries like China and Africa.

Human Immunodeficiency Virus infects cells of the immune system, destroying or severely impairing their function. HIV Is transmitted through unprotected sex, (vaginal, anal, oral), with an infected person. It is also transmitted through the transfusion of contaminated blood. Basically it is past with the introduction of human bodily fluids, including milk from a mother.

Acquired Immunodeficiency Syndrome, which applies to the most advanced stage of HIV. AIDS isn't the direct cause of death, but because of how it greatly impacts the immune system, the smallest cold can cause death. World AIDS Day, December 1, has become an incredibly important day throughout the world.

7. Diarrheal Diseases: 1.9 Million Deaths

Affects Africa (average of 130.3 per 1000,000 people), and India (132.7 per 100,000 people) the most and affects the greatest number of children under the age of 5. It is treatable and preventable, but many people who have it don't know, or can't afford the treatment. It is caused by the lack of safe drinking water and adequate sanitation and hygiene.

It kills about 760,000 children under the age of 5 and affects 1.7 billion people globally. In total, it was the cause of 1.9 million deaths in 2013, between children and adults.

6. Lung Cancer: 2 Million Deaths

A leading cause of death of people around the world, lung cancer is caused by multiple factors. It is the second most common cancer in the world after breast cancer. More than 8-10 cases of lung cancer are in people aged 60 or older, and the occurrence of lung cancer in Scotland is one of the highest. The lowest lung cancer rates are in Middle African countries.

Lung cancer has one of the lowest survival rates, as two-thirds of patients are diagnosed in too late of a stage when curative treatment is not possible. Around 30% of diagnosed people survive at least one year after diagnosis, and more than three/quarters of people who die from this cancer are 65 or over. Around 2 million people died worldwide in 2013.

The link between tobacco and cancer was established over 50 years ago, and smoking causes more than 4 in 5 lung cancers in the UK. Smoking, secondhand smoking, occupational exposures (such as asbestos), exposure to radon when you are a smoker increases your chances, and diesel exhaust. Poor diet is also a contributing factor.

5. COPD: 3.4 Million Deaths

Chronic Obstructive Pulmonary Disease is a long-term lung disease often caused by smoking. It is a life-threatening lung disease that interferes with normal breathing and an estimated 70 million people have COPD worldwide. Approximately 3.4 million people died this past year because of this serious lung blockage, and total deaths are expected to increase 30% over the next 10 years.

COPD is a lung disease that is characterized by the persistent blockage of airflow from the lungs. It is not fully reversible if treated, and chronic bronchitis and emphysema are now included with COPD.

Symptoms include: shortness of breath, a mix of saliva and mucus in the airway (abnormal sputum), and chronic coughing. It is not curable, but can be helped with various forms of treatment. Certain medicines that help dilate the airways are often used to help people have an easier time.

4. Lower Respiratory Infections: 3.4 Million Deaths

These infections include pneumonia, lung abscesses, and acute bronchitis. They are the leading causes of 3.4 million deaths around the world, which occurred mainly in children. Influenza also falls under this category.

Bronchitis can be acute or chronic, as well as bacterial or viral. It affects over 40 per 1000 adults each year, and consists of extreme inflammation of the major bronchi and trachea. Pneumonia occurs in a variety of situations and treatment can vary as well. It is most often caused by bacteria and is extremely dangerous with a mortality rate of 25%. Both of them can usually be cured with antibiotics, but they are very dangerous for elderly and those with immune deficiencies such as those with AIDS.

3. Diabetes: 3.5 Million Deaths

About 347 million people in the world suffer from diabetes and 3.5 million people died in 2013. Diabetes in Africa is especially problematic as a large portion of the population has diabetes, but 80% of those go undiagnosed. There are a few different types of diabetes:

Type 1: body's failure to produce sufficient amounts of insulin. Approximately 15% with diabetes has Type 1 and always need insulin treatments.

Type 2: body's resistance to insulin, often caused by normal or increases levels of circulating insulin. 85% have this type of diabetes and usually presents itself in people 30 years or older, but can show up earlier.

Gestational Diabetes: pregnant women who have never had diabetes before, but have high blood glucose levels during pregnancy are said to have this type. It can become Type 2 diabetes and affects about 4% of pregnant women.

2. Cerebrovascular Diseases: 6.2 Million Deaths

Stroke caused the death of 6.2 million people and tends to be higher in African-Americans. It is caused by the rapid loss of brain function due to a disturbance in the blood supply. This can be caused by lack of blood flow because of a blockage, or a hemorrhage. As a result the affected area of the brain cannot function, which can cause many serious problems later, such as lack of limb movement, or an inability to see.

A stroke is a medical emergency that can end with permanent neurological damage or death. Risk factors include old age, high blood pressure, previous history with strokes, diabetes, tobacco smoking, high cholesterol, and atrial fibrillation. It is the second most common and leading cause of death around the world.

About 87% of all strokes are caused by ischemia (hemorrhagic transformation). A hemorrhage is the accumulation of blood anywhere within the skull, and can be inside the brain or outside. It is unclear how many hemorrhages cause a stroke.

1. Ischaemic Heart Disease: 7 Million Deaths

IHD is the main contributing factor behind 7 million deaths around the world. Ischemia is when blood that normally flows to a part of the brain is temporarily restricted. When this happens to the heart it is called Cardiac Ischemia. The sudden restriction of blood going to the heart causes chest pain, or angina, which is actually a warning sign that something bad is about to happen. However, sometimes angina does not happen; this is called a silent heart attack. It is also very easy to mistake some lesser symptoms for heartburn and continue on with the day. About 25% of heart attacks are silent which is often why so many people die. People beyond the age of 60 are most affected, and much like the stroke, if you have history with having heart attacks, you are most likely to get them again.

**

51

13 SIERRA LEONE RED CROSS EMERGENCY PLAN OF ACTION: EBOLA VIRUS DISEASE

A. Situation analysis

Description of the disaster

In March, an outbreak of Ebola virus disease (EVD) was detected in Guinea close to the borders of Sierra Leone and Liberia. At that time, the Sierra Leone Ministry of Health and Sanitation established a National Ebola Taskforce to coordinate activities to prevent and prepare for the detection of EVD in the country. The Sierra Leone Red Cross Society (SLRCS) has played a key part in these activities, with training of volunteers and dissemination of information in the seven priority districts of Bombali, Kailahun, Kenema, Koinadugu, Kono, and Western rural/urban (Freetown). Information on Ebola awareness has been communicated at all levels of society using a variety of formats and methods: printed educational materials, radio jingles and talk shows, TERA messaging, use social media, and house-to-house visits.

On 26 May, the Ministry of Health and Sanitation announced that the first case of EVD had been detected in Sierra Leone. Soon after, a further seven cases were identified. All of these early cases resided in the Kissi Teng Chiefdom which forms the easternmost part of Kailahun District. All eight persons had attended the funeral of a traditional healer in Guinea. Difficulties in accessing communities to track potential contacts, alongside insufficient infrastructure to deal with the rapidly increasing caseload, make it difficult to ascertain precisely the evolution of the outbreak. The number of reported cases and deaths, contacts under medical observation and the number of laboratory results are in constant flux.

On 11 June, the President of Sierra Leone declared that Kailahun was in a state of emergency. Since this announcement, military personnel have been placed on access points to screen people moving in and out of the district for fever. Schools and other institution of learning remain closed, quarantining of more districts, stay-at-home approach, vigorous monitoring of commuters by temperature checking and hand washing along the main roads from Freetown to the countryside.

The incidence of Ebola virus disease in Sierra Leone continues to remain very high and spreading far and wide, with almost 200 new cases reported in the past weeks. Ebola cases and deaths in Sierra Leone continue to escalate with an upsurge in the number of new confirmed cases reported in the past few weeks. The capital, Freetown, now seems to be the new hotspot of the Ebola crisis with an increase in cases reported over the last few weeks. The rate of transmission in Freetown and main cities are also spiking high with reports of dead bodies littering the streets of Freetown. Transmission in Kailahun and Kenema is relatively stable, where the Red Cross presence is highly visible. There has been an increase in the number of new cases reported in the districts of Bo, Bombali, and Port Loko. The district of Koinadugu, which had been Ebola free, reported its first cases recently.

The rate of infections of the virus among healthcare workers in the country is at an alarming degree with considerable numbers of government hospitals recording low staff with empty hospital beds. It's gratifying to note no Red Cross personnel has been infected since the start of clinical case management/dead body management. The Red Cross will continue to instill discipline in the minds of all volunteers and staff involved, continue to conduct more training and monitoring of safe and dignified burials in areas where the national society is operational.

The daily reclassification of cases by the Sierra Leone Ministry of Health and Sanitation reveal a cumulative number of laboratory confirmed cases of 2,977 and 932 confirmed deaths, corresponding to a case fatality rate of 31.3% as of 14 October 2014.

The IFRC Ebola Treatment Centre (ETC) in Kenema commenced formal operation in September 13, 2014 with a capacity of 60 beds. The ETC has currently recorded 114 admissions, recorded 43 deaths, discharged 31 and transferred 8. The operation is supported by 124 locally hired nurses, clinicians, WatSan and auxiliary staff with about 12 ERU (international staff) as reported on 22 October.

Summary of the current response
Since the first alert that suspected cases could have crossed the border, SLRCS has been coordinating its activities with the Ministry of Health and Sanitation (MoHS). In response to the EVD outbreak in Sierra Leone, the IFRC continues to provide technical and financial support to the National Society.

Following the confirmation of cases in Guinea on March 28 2014, the IFRC allocated CHF 113,217 from its Disaster Relief Emergency Fund (DREF) for Ebola Preparedness activities in Sierra Leone. Following the confirmation of cases within the borders of Sierra Leone, the DREF allocation was converted into a start-up loan for the Emergency Appeal operation launched on 26 June 2014.

On 1 April, the Ministry of Health and Sanitation formally requested SLRCS to lead on awareness and social mobilization campaigns at the county level based on its large team of volunteers on the ground. Later, a Memorandum of Understanding between government and National Society was signed regarding safe and dignified burials in Kailahun. A further meeting was held with the Ministry of Health and Sanitation in which assistance was requested for volunteers to support contact tracing and psychosocial support activities. Since the initial confirmation of cases, the government has responded with the following activities:
- Provision of free treatment for EVD cases
- Intensification of community sensitization activities
- Distribution of Personal Protective Equipment to affected regions
- Strengthening of surveillance
- Development of a case management protocol
- Training of healthcare workers to staff isolation rooms and treatment centres

Health Ministers and technical staff from 11 countries, representatives from IFRC, MSF, WHO and key international partner organizations met in an Emergency Ministerial meeting in Accra, Ghana 2 and 3 July to address the ongoing EVD outbreak in West Africa. After updates and country and field experiences were shared, they agreed on a strategy for an accelerated operational response to control the outbreak. Since then, WHO opened a regional control center in Conakry, Guinea, and urged governments to work with religious and community leaders to improve awareness and understanding of EVD.

Until the outbreak, the IFRC did not have representation in the country and had been supporting SLRCS through its regional office for West Africa in Cote d'Ivoire. IFRC has a coordination hub currently based in Conakry, Guinea which is coordinating the whole response in the affected countries. Before the confirmation of cases in Sierra Leone, regional staff were deployed to support the SLRCS in preparedness activities. As the situation deteriorated and the National Society initiated response to active cases, an IFRC Field Assessment and Coordination Team (FACT) was deployed and arrived in Freetown in early June, followed by staff from the Basic Health Care ERU and IT/Telecomm Emergency Response Units.

IFRC has set up offices in Freetown, a base in Kailahun and the ETC in Kenema. In relation to the scaling up, IFRC is supporting the NS in implementing activities outlined in all the pillars in five other districts, namely, Bo, Bombali, Kenema, Port Loko, Western Area Rural and Urban and plans to further extend its operations in Moyamba, Tonkilili, Pujehum and Kambia.

DBM, contact tracing, PSS, and social mobilization have been implemented, in all the eleven operational areas and clinical management in the IFRC ETC in Kenema. To date, the IFRC Ebola operation has achieved the following;

- **433** safe and dignified burials.
- **820** volunteers trained and active in the Ebola operation.
- **17,470** contacts traced and followed up by the Red Cross

volunteers
- **1,352** houses and public facilities disinfected
- **774,348** people reached through door to door social mobilisation campaigns
- **2,090** people received psychosocial support and re-integrated back into the community after treatment
- **144** patients treated at the Red Cross treatment centre in Kenema.
- Over **7 million** SMS on Ebola prevention sent across the country.
- Millions of people have been reached with Ebola prevention and awareness through radio dramas and the weekly live one-hour radio call-in show for questions and answers about Ebola aired on a national radio station.
- Pre-positioning of personal protective equipment and related training on their proper use and disposal;
- Interagency coordination through the National Task Force and at the field level in 10 districts.

The IFRC has established a regional Ebola response and preparedness coordination function through its Ebola Management Unit in Conakry, Guinea. The unit carries out outbreak-wide data collection and analysis, knowledge management, cross-border collaboration, resource mobilization and consistent effective preparedness and response and provides coordination at strategic level.

Interagency Coordination
The SLRCS is a member the National Ebola Taskforce with the Ministry of Health, World Health Organization and NGO partners including Médecins Sans Frontières, Save the Children and Action Contre la Faime. It is also a member of the taskforces established at a district level and daily coordination meetings take place in Kailahun under joint MoHS/WHO leadership. Under the national taskforce are five pillars:

1. laboratories and surveillance;
2. case management,
3. social mobilization,

4. logistics
5. coordination.

The same technical coordination structures have been established in Kailahun and each of these groups meet twice a week. Updates on the epidemiological situation are provided at the taskforce meetings and are also published on the Ministry of Health and Sanitation's Facebook page and the WHO Global Alert and Response website.

Risk Assessment

Initial hopes that the outbreak could be contained within Kailahun have subsided as cases have now been reported in all 13 districts including Koinadugu which had until recently been Ebola free. In addition, new chains of cases may emerge with no known contacts or from sources outside Sierra Leone. The capacity of the Ministry of Health and Sanitation to identify and isolate cases has proven insufficient. MSF has also warned that it is facing difficulties in scaling up to needs, as it is already taking care of most of the current caseload.

It is also possible that the outbreak, or the measures implemented to control the outbreak, could lead to tensions and social unrest. While not on a scale such as what has been happening in neighbouring Guinea, isolated attacks have taken place against MoHS ambulances in the course of their Ebola-related activities, perpetrated by angry community members.

On 10 June, the President of Sierra Leone announced a state of emergency in Kailahun with a number of effects:
1. Closure of schools
2. Prohibition of large gatherings
3. Burials without approval of the District Health Medical Team have been prohibited
4. Quarantining of districts

People moving into or out of Kailahun Kenema, Bombali, Port Loko and Moyemba must be screened by volunteers who take their temperature, look for symptoms of the disease under supervision of the military. Vehicles in these areas have also been restricted to move between 9 AM to 5 PM.

5. Introduction of a "Stay-at-home" campaign as a way of containing the outbreak

Organisational risk

EVD is a highly infectious disease. There is risk that Red Cross staff and volunteers operating in affected communities could contract the disease, particularly in the course of DBM activities. The IFRC's global volunteer insurance only provides coverage in case of accidents, but not from diseases like Ebola. SLRCS and IFRC are currently looking at additional coverage options in country to provide complementary insurance to its staff and volunteers.

Needs analysis

Based on an assessment conducted in June by FACT team and on the deteriorating situation since, the following needs have been identified:

1.Social mobilization and Beneficiary communication.

Despite progress, knowledge of Ebola virus disease and mode of transmission remains limited within the population and rumours and misconceptions regarding the mode of transmission (or even outright denial) linger. Due to the highly infectious nature of the disease many people are fearful and stigma remains high. Despite the major efforts deployed so far in awareness raising and education, there is still a significant need to scale these up as the main obstacle to effective patient identification, contact tracing and reintegration remains ignorance.

The needs assessment (including preliminary results of the Rapid Mobile-Phone based survey) identified a number of information gaps that could be contributing to disease transmission. There is also a lack of awareness that dead bodies are a significant source of transmission. Several people expressed that they would not believe EVD existed until they had seen it themselves.

There are also specific behavioural issues that could contribute to the spread of the disease and that could be specifically addressed. For example, dead bodies are often transported on motorcycles, held between the driver and a relative. There are also important cultural reasons why families wish to see the body of a relative prior to their burial. The traditional funeral rituals in many communities involve substantial contact with the deceased person.

To date, the social mobilization strategy has started to address the potential stigma that individuals and families affected by EVD may experience.

Overall, there is a need to regularly review the key messages to ensure they are relevant to the current situation and meet the information needs of the community. It will be important to specifically address perceptions about EVD that lead to stigmatisation of families affected by the disease.

Innovative approaches need to be expanded in order to effectively disseminate information to communities and target those at highest risk, as well as communities where the most vulnerable are to be found. It is known that women are disproportionately represented in this outbreak, most likely because they tend to care for sick family members.

Discharged patients, both Ebola survivors and those tested Ebola negative also face substantial risk of stigmatization and rejection and therefore targeting their families and communities is vital both before and after discharge.

Based on the results from the EVD Knowledge, Attitudes and Practices survey done through a Rapid Mobile-Phone approach, we know that most people get their information through: friends and neighbours, radio, health centre or health workers and Red Cross volunteers or staff (their most trusted source). Radio programmes as a way of disseminating messages should especially be used since 90% of the people have access to them. Radio Moa and Sierra Leone Red Cross Society are the two main radio stations that people listen to in the eastern districts.

Given that the worst affected chiefdoms have strong cultural ties to people in the neighbouring districts in Guinea and Liberia, there is an ongoing need to ensure communication with this group is coordinated across all three countries and that messages targeting this group are consistent.

Community-based solutions on how we conquer Ebola are at the forefront of the response. As much as we try to provide solutions, it will be the communities who are the main implementers and will play a joint role as frontline responders.

Establishing processes within established communication networks and communities that allow the population to clearly voice their understanding of the issues and provide feedback will build stronger trust and a more community-led solution.

Approaches that emphasize community strengthening and participation, as well as partnership building between communities and participating agencies have proven to be more effective than top-down communication interventions.

These approaches go beyond educating people about health risks. They facilitate local dialogue and relationships that empower people to abandon unhealthy traditional practices and harmful norms, building more community resilience to respond to the impacts of disease outbreaks. Embedded in the DBM Teams will be a Beneficiary Communication/Community Engagement (BC/CE) volunteer tasked with the process of engaging with the community during the body removal process. The BC/CE volunteer will utilize the time during the process to talk with the community about their understanding of the DBM process, their understanding of Ebola in general and answer any questions the community members may have. There will also be an opportunity to provide IEC materials. The BC/CE volunteer will also be tasked with gathering information, using a set of questions within the RAMP system, a mobile phone data-gathering tool. The information will allow the RC to gather information that will allow us to assess the current situations and perceptions in the communities as well as gathering data about the family and the affected person. The process will strengthen our accountability to the community and families by providing safe and dignified burials and through the collection of data enable us to provide information relating to the affected persons' Ebola status and location of burial.

2. Safe and Dignified Burials and Disinfection

As the caseload increased and the MoHS resources proved insufficient to respond, the SLRCS received an official request from the government on 6 July to engage in the management of dead bodies, burials and disinfection of houses. This being a new technical area of intervention for the National Society, the IFRC facilitated contact with MSF and WHO to organise training on safe practice and procedures.

A total of fourteen volunteers were therefore trained in safe and dignified burials on the 11th of July. The training continued for 3 days, after which the team became ready to support the response in transport of the corpse, disinfection and burials. In some cases, potentially contaminated items belonging to infected patients will need to be destroyed. In these instances, the burial teams will refer the families to the PSS volunteers accompanying the deceased person's relatives for them to provide a support package (hygiene kit, mattress etc.)

Chlorine and PPE kits continue to be short in supply. One of the main risks of transmissions comes from dead bodies.

Another high risk of contamination comes from traditional burial practices, where relatives touch and wash the body of the deceased family member, then share a meal together. Proper supervision of the burial practices, accompanied with active education and awareness activities and engagement from religious leaders, is a high priority to reduce the risk of transmission during burials.

It also appears that the homes of many confirmed cases are not being disinfected. Where this takes place, there is a need to provide support to those whose possessions have to be destroyed.

Additional efforts must also be made to ensure that houses are properly disinfected to eliminate the risk of further contamination of family members.

As the caseload continues to increase and spread to new districts, IFRC, through the revised plan, will significantly increase the safe and dignified burial team from the initial 3 teams to 29 teams across the country. In the capital, Freetown, the National Society has mobilized about 100 volunteers for collection and burial of human remains inside Freetown where the caseload (Ebola death) is overwhelming.

In order to provide wider coverage and speed, currently, ten SLRCS burial teams have been established in Freetown alone (6 in Urban and 4 team in Rural Freetown). It is envisaged that within a couple of weeks all teams will be adequately trained, fully equipped and logistically strong to carry out the activities in assigned areas in Freetown. New cadre of volunteers shall constitute these teams and better-quality community engagement and data collection. The national society continues to enjoy trust with local authorities/communities and ensuring the safety and security of its volunteers to carry out their various tasks.

3. Psychosocial Support

There is no organization currently addressing PSS needs related to the EVD outbreak in the affected areas. Nevertheless, a range of psychosocial needs have been identified in EVD outbreaks in Guinea, Liberia and Uganda.

Fear of Ebola and stigmatization of those affected and others has both short and long-term effects. In the short-term, fear and stigmatization influences help-seeking behaviour, i.e. the belief that Ebola always kills and that sick people are dangerous makes people helpless and fearful when faced with disease. This also stigmatizes health workers as they are seen to be potentially dangerous and contagious.

In the long term the stigma on affected individuals and families is likely to linger and health care workers and volunteers working with Ebola have experienced significant, lasting stigmatization.

Volunteers, many of whom will be living in affected communities, are likely to be under great stress during the epidemic. Therefore, close supervision, psychosocial support and organizational recognition for volunteers is a vital component of the response.

The development and delivery of one day training for SLRC volunteers in community mobilisation and PSS is essential to get the right Ebola messages and right preventive and case management methods through. The training is to update and refresh the knowledge on Ebola. Information about contact tracing and dead body management is essential as well to alleviate the fear and stigma.

4. Surveillance, Case Identification and Contact Management

Each district has a government surveillance team. In Kailahun, for example, there are currently two to three teams of 3 people in each. The actual need is estimated to be eight teams of 4 people. Given the rapidly increasing number of cases, these teams do not have the capacity to follow-up on all alerts in a timely manner, monitor contacts and collect accurate epidemiological data.

The current surveillance system relies mainly on sick people identifying themselves or others to the healthcare system. However, in some communities, ill people have been reluctant to seek help from healthcare workers. Hence, it is likely that cases are not being notified and managed. Early identification and isolation of cases as well as follow-up of case contact is critical to control of the outbreak, so this area continues to be a critical need.

The expanded appeal will train 330 volunteers in all the 11 branches for surveillance and contact tracing of suspected, probable and confirmed cases, then undertake contact tracing and follow-up activities by volunteers in communities, using infra-red thermometers and reporting regularly on contact tracing using mobile phones.

5. Case management

Given the increase in Ebola caseload and geographical spread of cases the number of ETC is increasing. Units are now functioning in Kailahun, Kenema (IFRC), Bo, Connaught, Hastings-Freetown, Laka, 34 Military hospital, Macauly, PCMH and Rokupa. Further units are planned in all affected districts, including a large unit in Port Loko. Given the gap in available ETC beds and case numbers, a change of strategy is being proposed that includes smaller centres of 5 to 10 beds managed by community health workers implementing full PPE and IPC standards. Current planning for this is dynamic, but an estimated 200 units are being proposed.

A change in isolation management will affect all other activities, in terms of how they are implemented and how they engage in communication, coordination and collaboration with these units. Continual assessment will be needed to assess the Infection Prevention Control levels in each centre and recommendations on how NS volunteers can engage with them are agreed.

The IFRC managed ETC in Kenema has been providing clinical case management for Ebola cases since 5th September. The planned bed capacity of 60 beds should be fully realised by the end of October. Difficulties in attracting enough international staff with the right profiles in the initial stages have delayed the scale up to full capacity. However new initiatives in expanding the recruitment base and pre-deployment trainings with support of a Geneva based team has increased the supply of HR and will ensure the functioning of the unit going forward.

6. Regional preparedness, coordination and response

This epidemic is the first time that EVD has occurred in West Africa. The epidemic has presented particular challenges with a number of widely dispersed clusters, some affecting urban areas, spreading across borders. Due to the regional nature of the outbreak, there is a need for the IFRC to work with the concerned National Societies to develop a regional preparedness and response plan, ensure strategic coordination between the three country operations and be prepared to deal with escalation to other countries should it become necessary.

B. Operational strategy and plan

Overall objective
Contribute to the reduction of mortality and morbidity related to the Ebola virus disease in Sierra Leone through awareness messaging, safe and dignified burials, contact tracing, social mobilization provide psychosocial support and case management/treatment to those affected.

Proposed strategy
Given the unprecedented and extensive spread of EVD in the country and main cities in particular it is imperative to do more in breaking the chain of transmission. Three districts have recently been quarantined due to the surge in caseloads, bringing the total number of quarantined districts to five. Koinadugu District, which had been Ebola free, has recently reported more than 15 cases. The main cities continue to report spikes, with dead bodies littering the streets of Freetown.

SLRCS will undertake the appropriate and efficient management of dead bodies in all the ten districts. This will include collection of corpses from homes, morgues, and even with a PSS approach, ensuring cultural practices when possible and care for families when needed, undertake safe and dignified burials, and the disinfection of contaminated homes and areas.

The services will be carried out by 224 adequately trained and well-equipped SLRCS volunteers organized into teams comprising: four (4) stretcher-bearers, two (2) sprayers, one (1) dresser, and one (1) beneficiary communication volunteer.

Each team of 10 is completed with 2 staff drivers (1 pick-up single cabin for dead bodies and one hardtop to transport the burial team). Training of these teams has commenced and is expected to be completed within two weeks, after which all DBM teams shall be fully operational. All dead body management (DBM) teams will undergo quality assurance checks by SLRCS Dead Body supervisors and external partners/experts on a regular basis, in order to ensure safety.

The SLRCS is strategically placed to intervene at the household level through its extensive network of active volunteers.

The national society will mobilize 1,854 active volunteers supported by over 70 staff in the 11 operational areas within the 10 Branches/Districts. The national society has recently recruited 34 field staff with more than 25 drivers who have been exclusively employed for the Ebola response. Another set of 20 staff is expected to be recruited for the 4 branches/districts considered as new Ebola hotspots.

SLRCS Dead Body Management Supervisors at its national headquarters will coordinate and supervise the collection of corpses and perform safe and dignified burials under the overall management of the National Ebola Coordinator and a highly experienced Dead Body Management Supervisor at headquarters with specifically identified DBM officer in each of the branches, whilst the IFRC ensures longer-term oversight and management of the operation with additional and specialised human resources providing technical support.

Freetown alone has 10 teams and has started collecting bodies. Within a time span of two days more than 30 bodies have been collected and buried. The national society DBM Hotline telephone number 300 has been re-activated and has started receiving calls and responding accordingly.

DBM Volunteers of the national society in particular continue to be rejected by their own families, friends and even communities. Alternative strategies are being designed to alleviate the conditions of affected volunteers. These include explicit PSS sessions with such families, allocation of rooms for DMB volunteers, increasing their daily incentives, complementary insurance packages, and special family allowances in case of death, etc. The national society will continue to strive harder in maintaining the zero fatality rate for DBM and other teams operating in the country.

Embedded in the DBM Teams will be a Beneficiary Communication / Community Engagement (BC/CE) volunteer tasked with the process of engaging with the community during the body removal process. The BC/CE volunteer will utilize the time during the process to talk with the community about their understanding of the DBM process, their understanding of Ebola in general and answer any questions the community members may have.

There will also be an opportunity to provide IEC materials. The BC/CE volunteer will also be tasked with gathering information using a set of questions within the RAMP system, a mobile phone data-gathering tool. The information will allow the RC to gatherer information that will allow us to assess the current situations and perceptions in the communities as well as gathering data about the family and the affected person.

The process will strengthen our accountability to the community and families by providing safe and dignified burials and through the collection of data enable us to provide information relating to the affected persons Ebola status and location of burial.

Community based solutions to how we conquer Ebola are at the forefront of the response. As much as we try to provide solutions, it will be the communities who are the main implementers and will play a joint role as frontline responders.

Establishing processes within established communication networks and communities that allow the population to clearly voice their understanding of the issues and provide feedback will build stronger trust and a more community-led solution.

Approaches that emphasize community strengthening and participation, as well as partnership building between communities and participating agencies, have proven to be more effective than top-down communication interventions.

These approaches go beyond educating people about health risks. They facilitate local dialogue and relationships that empower people to abandon unhealthy traditional practices and harmful norms, building more community resilience to respond to the impacts of disease outbreaks.

The National Society supports the Government in drafting the Sierra Leone Emergency Management Program Standard Operating Procedure for Safe, Dignified Medical Burials.

Social mobilisation activities shall be implemented in 113 chiefdoms focusing on mass sensitisation and health/sanitation campaigns with established Ebola information kiosks and hand washing stations and supply of soaps to vulnerable communities. PSS support the discharged patients to reintegrate back to their communities and in contract training patients who turn out to be negative shall be keenly followed-up 21 days by volunteers who shall be provided with telephones and air time to give feedback and each branch allocated with a vehicle (one hard top) to carry out these activities.

Social mobilisation and recent incorporated beneficiary communication, robust community engagement and data collection, as well as surveillance and contact tracing, and psychological support service are integral activities for the national society in undertaking all of its operational areas. Officers have been recruited to coordinate the implementation of these activities in each of the districts in close coordination and partnership with The Ministry of Health and Sanitation as part of its mandate and auxiliary role, MSH/Districts Health Management Teams and WHO and relevant stakeholders.

The national society diverts its focus on response to the Ebola operations overstretching its meagre resources. Huge funds are utilised in rental costs/hiring both in fleet and warehousing. Therefore, the construction of a central warehouse and two mini-regional warehouses are seen as a better alternative and a capacity development aspect of the national society when the operation is terminated.

Despite efforts to contain it, the outbreak has continued to spread and the resources deployed so far in the response –by the country's authorities, the RC/RC Movement, MSF and other partners- are proving insufficient.

Most recently, in regards to the ERU request for treatment response at the Kenema Hospital, the need to scale up is mostly manifested in clinical staff and logistics, in addition to needs initially proposed through the Emergency Appeal launched in June, including expansion of volunteer mobilization in education, awareness raising and social mobilization, contact tracing and surveillance, PSS support and dead body management, supervision of burials and disinfection of houses.

The revised plan of action will build on the activities already being conducted in these districts to enhance the response to EVD and focus on the needs of Kenema Hospital. In addition to clinical staff, the ERU requested logistical, finance and administrative support.

The SLRCS has recruited a National Ebola Coordinator based at HQ in Freetown and at branch level District Operation Managers, DBM Coordinators and Community Engagement Officers, have begun to be recruited. To date, some 120 officers have been recruited. Their responsibilities will be devoted exclusively to the Ebola response operation. At HQ, a Rapid Response/ Mobile Team will be established.

Social Mobilisation, Contact Tracing and PSS will be carried out nationally, in all the 13 districts. 550 volunteers in all districts will be trained in EVD signs and symptoms, prevention measures and referral mechanisms including personal protection. Special training will be conducted for 330 volunteers in Surveillance and Contact Tracing in all the 11 operation areas.

The following SLRCS branch offices will be fully operational (well-functional offices: internet facility, generators, IT equipment, vehicles, stationary and trained personnel) in Kailahun, Kenema,

Port Loko, Western Area, Bo and Bombali Districts. Six out of the thirteen districts in Sierra Leone will be fully operational in promoting community awareness, preventative hygiene measures and safe burials. The Dead Body Management teams will be allocated accommodation in each of the operational areas to enable them to recuperate; shower and rest as a considerable number of volunteers are exposed to rejection by their own families. A cook will be provided to help with their living arrangements.

To aim for a zero fatality rate for the volunteers and staff involved in DBM activities, their training in the use of PPE will be refreshed regularly (every six weeks) and will be subject to a quality assurance check by external specialists (MSF or WHO). All deaths in the hot-spots are considered Ebola related unless proven otherwise by laboratory tests, therefore the DBM teams conduct all burials if and when contacted by the District Health Management Team. This will require procurement of 5000 personnel protective kits and 5000 body bags.

The plan is to have at least 120 volunteers in each district engaged in hygiene promotion and community mobilization, contact tracing and surveillance, psychosocial support activities and dead body management. This will bring the number of volunteers involved in the operation to a total of 2,188 countrywide.

The National Society will procure 20 infra-red thermometers for use in all its offices throughout the country, with special volunteers/staff to be trained on the usage of this equipment.

Education, awareness and social mobilization are the most effective means to tackle the disease as this combination increases reporting of sick people to seek early medical attention and facilitates access for medical personnel and contact tracers to communities. Proper contact tracing and surveillance allows for an informed response and detection of potential cases, while the timely management of dead bodies, proper and supervised burial practices and disinfection are the most effective way to prevent further propagation.

As contact tracing and surveillance systems improve, the SLRC will be utilizing this information to identify affected villages for target intervention to reduce transmission. Utilizing surveillance data that records where cases and contacts are, will allow specific villages at risk of high rates of transmission to be targeted for prevention education, contact tracing and alert notification.

By ensuring those who are most at risk understand how to prevent further transmission, when and why they should come to the hospital we can reduce the amount of transmission within these communities. This includes even targeting down to the household level, where there is heavy transmission and clusters of cases. Social mobilization and health education should be implemented using a PSS approach targeting the effected community to limit next generation transmission and ensure community compliance.

In reality this means, volunteers need cross- training in PSS and social mobilization and both sides should be working as one team. The work plan for the day should be guided by the surveillance and contact tracing data that would indicate specific clusters of cases. This will require more technical engagement and oversight as well as have implications on logistics as teams will need to move to the cases rather than just work in their specific areas.

Rapid response:
Given the limited funds available for further scale up, it is imperative that we move to areas of new transmission quickly to scale up key activities including contact tracing, dead body management and community engagement. A rapid response to newly affected areas will limit transmission and allow for localised cases to be contained. All SLRC districts have been trained and are implementing key prevention activities. If a confirmed case is registered in a district, and gaps in response capacity are identified, the rapid response team from Freetown will be deployed. The objective of this team is to quickly implement key activities in a safe and controlled way and undertake training, capacity building and supervision of new teams that are established in response to the new cases. This will also assist in sharing learning and best

practices across districts.

Prevention and disease surveillance:
All districts without cases will continue social mobilisation and active disease surveillance to ensure any cases are rapidly identified and communities understand the need to come forward as soon as possible. This activity is important and should be prioritised despite current constraints, as it will stop further geographical spread of cases. This revision of the strategy will require more technical engagement and oversight as well, as it has implications on logistics.

Teams will need to move to the cases rather than work in their specific areas. Engagement with available technical advisors on the ground both internally, and through agencies such as CDC and WHO will provide the technical analysis needed to target transmission hot spots ensuring we are having maximum impact on transmission changes and the evolution of the epidemic.

Prevention and Disease Surveillance team:
Will provide support to non-infected or cleared districts to ensure disease surveillance. The Rapid Response Team (Mobile Team) at SLRCS national headquarters consisting of a doctor/nurse, DBM specialist, Contact Tracing specialist and allocated with a vehicle and a driver will respond to spikes/alerts within 48 hours.

Definitions of Activities:

Community Engagement: Social mobilization will include discussions and interactions with communities to educate them about Ebola and to ensure that they are implementing the key messages to prevent and contain Ebola. It also involves passive contact tracing, meaning, if cases are found at the community level they will be referred or notified. This is done using a PSS approach. Social mobilization should include a full communication plan and rumour management strategy.

Alert and contact team: Active case follow up with a PSS approach will involve volunteers who will be assigned specific contacts to follow up for 21 days. Social mobilization occurs as part of the follow up to educate families on prevention and control. A PSS approach ensures improved engagement and compliance.

Active PSS: This includes targeted PSS activities including grief management and community re-entry.

Dead Body Management: Involves collection of bodies from the communities of clinical facilities for burial with a PSS approach, ensuring cultural practices when possible and care for families when needed.

The epidemic 'frontline' – a focus of all key activities in districts that have large amounts of active transmission. This includes Kenema, Kailahun, and Western district. This will include contributing to case management in Kenema. In regards to the response initially proposed through the Revised Emergency Appeal launched in September the need for further scale up is most manifest in the expansion of volunteer mobilization in safe and dignified burials activities, education, awareness raising and social mobilization, contact tracing and surveillance and PSS support. The revised strategy also includes a new area of intervention in dead body management, supervision of burials and disinfection of houses.

Beneficiary selection

In addition to having a national range, and based on the assessments carried out and indications provided by the Ministry of Health and Sanitation, the plan of action emphasises high risk groups and opinion leaders such as:
- Women's groups and associations
- Bike riders and drivers
- Schools
- Religious and traditional healer leaders
- Health workers
- Ebola patients

Special attention will be given to women and women's groups

since this is an especially vulnerable group. To date, MoHS reports indicate that 59% of the people affected by EVD are women. The health workers affected have been mainly women and women are the ones that take care of their sick family members and relatives. They are also the ones that care for the body of the person that has died, which is highly infectious if not dealt with properly.

Progress of implementation to date

The Sierra Leone Red Cross Society has been implementing its response along the following five pillars:

1. Education, awareness raising and social mobilization

A widespread program of community sensitization was undertaken during the preparation phase funded under the DREF using a set of 13 key messages approved by the Ministry of Health and Sanitation. The National Society played a major role in the sensitization program, training 15 volunteers in six districts (Freetown and the five districts that border Guinea) on EVD, including the signs and symptoms, mode of transmission and what people should do if they become sick. In Kailahun, the Programme Administrator arranged for an additional 35 volunteers to be trained to make a total of 50.

Following their training, the volunteers have conducted sensitization activities in all targeted districts.

400 volunteers have been identified and been trained in awareness creation and sensitization in all the areas of operation. They have been carrying out sensitization and awareness session for women's groups, bikers union, religious congregations and disabled people (blind, amputees, polio patients and war wounded).

A Red Cross Drama Group has on several occasions performed a play were they, through acting, address issues around Ebola such as stigma, myths and awareness. The Drama has become high in demand and is being used in many trainings in Kailahun District, as it generates a lot of questions and discussions from the audience after each performance.

401 leaders from various community networks participated in three days of awareness raising communication organized by the Red Cross, MSF and the MoHS. These included Paramount Chiefs, Section Chiefs, Speaker Mammy Queens Youth Leaders, Chiefdom Soweis, Religious leaders, Ward Councillors, Children representatives, Bike Riders, Traders and Drivers' Union. At the end of the day, these leaders and opinion-makers drafted plans of action to disseminate Ebola related messaging to their respective networks.

IEC material has been prepared and distributed to the branches in and the volunteers and ERU delegates have participated in local radio shows where the listeners could call in to ask questions.

People have been reached through house-to-house awareness visits in Kailahun while most households have received visits from the SLRCS in Kenema.

On 26.06 and 30.06, over 106 people from women's groups in Kailahun participated in an awareness-raising workshop. This specific group was targeted because women, as traditional caregivers, are more exposed to the virus and constitute 60% of the affected population.

Over 20,000 people have been reached directly so far by the SLRCS, over 193 communities in six districts.

The SLRCS is using the TERA (Trilogy Emergency Relief Application) SMS system to reach hundreds of thousands of people with simple, practical advice on preventing and responding to Ebola, as well as information to counteract the myths and stigma surrounding the disease. The TERA system gives SLRCS the capacity to target SMS to specific geographical locations, meaning the information received by people can be tailored to their actual situation and needs, and therefore more relevant and likely to have an impact.

The system can also ask questions and accept answers back,

allowing it to be used for simple surveys. Since the outbreak of the Ebola epidemic SLRCS has sent more than 289,000 SMS to people in affected areas, increasing the reach and impact of health activities beyond those who can be reached face to face. SMS is also a safe means of reaching people remotely, when face-to-face contact is a risk for volunteers. While the SMS themselves are free to send, there are technical support fees and some running costs, which are included in the appeal budget.

In early July, cases started to appear in Bo, the second largest city in Sierra Leone. In response, two of the ERU hygiene promoters redeployed there to do an awareness and sensitization training for 30 volunteers.

2. Surveillance, case identification and contact management
A total of 400 volunteers have been trained in contact tracing in all the response districts . The PSS delegate has participated in the trainings, conducted and supervised by the MoHS. These volunteers are part of the larger +200 group of volunteers managed and supervised by the MoHS.

The IFRC epidemiologist has assisted MoHS, WHO and MSF in data collection and management activities and to identify potential gaps in contact tracing and supported the SLRCS to develop a strategy for monitoring the daily activities of the Red Cross volunteers engaged in contact tracing.

SLRCS will continue to have volunteers attend the trainings and join the surveillance networks as they are expanded to other districts. The next two districts to be prioritized are Kenema and Bo.

3. Dead Body Management
As the caseload increased and the MoHS resources proved insufficient to respond, the SLRCS received an official request from the government on the 6 July to engage in the management of dead bodies, burials and disinfection of houses. This being a new technical area of intervention for the National Society, the IFRC facilitated contact with MSF and WHO to organise training on safe

practice and procedures.

A total of fourteen volunteers were therefore trained in Dead Body Management (DBM) on 11 July. To date, 224 volunteers are involved in the safe and dignified burials and disinfection activities. 433 burials have been conducted across the country with 1,352 houses and public spaces disinfected. As the number of Ebola deaths continue to soar, there is a growing need to expand the burial team.

The new plan is to have 29 Dead Body Management (DBM) teams across the country with each team comprising of 4 stretcher bearers, 2 sprayers, a communicator and a supervisor with two drivers and two vehicles (1 pick-up single cabin for dead bodies and one hard top to transport the burial team) in a branch.

4. Psychosocial Support
A Red Cross community-based psychosocial support (PSS) intervention is being organized in Kailahun district for vulnerable groups including vulnerable hospitalized and discharged patients (Ebola survivors and Ebola negative) and families affected by Ebola (separated, bereaved, etc.).

In addition, the psychosocial support team may support with community dialogue and reintegration, preparing the ground for activities of other RC teams and partners (surveillance, case management and burial) and provide targeted sensitization in hot spots.

The PSS intervention is planned, coordinated and conducted in collaboration with Médecins Sans Frontières, Save the Children, Community Association for Psychosocial Support (CAPS) and the Children's Advocacy and Rehabilitation (CAR) centre of the SLRCS. The community based psychosocial intervention will be conducted by 400 volunteers.

The volunteers are receiving an initial one-day training on sensitization and psychosocial support and will receive monthly follow-up trainings, including case management and peer support sessions. Ongoing support will be provided through weekly supervision calls by trained counsellors from the CAR centre. The team will also include trained psychosocial counsellors from CAPS.

The counsellors may support the volunteers with the work in the communities, if necessary. The volunteers will also feedback any information on affected cases and developments in the community to the Branch Health Officer (BHO) at Kailahun branch. The BHO will also serve as the focal point for referrals of vulnerable beneficiaries from partners (Médecins Sans Frontières, Save the Children and others).

PSS volunteers will also be the focal points for families having had personal property items destroyed as part of the disinfection process, to replace those items with a standardized support package.

The information needs of the community will be regularly reviewed using a further survey, feedback from volunteers and community members and other media such as talkback radio. Messages will be updated to ensure these needs continue to be met. SLRCS will continue to seek new opportunities to access and influence communities and groups that have been hard to reach or are at high risk.

5. Regional preparedness, coordination and response
Resource mobilization remains a continuous challenge, especially for non-medical activities. Huge efforts are, however, put into ensuring funding for all five priority pillars. Without solid interventions within these we will not be able to stop the Ebola outbreak. Contact tracing, disinfection of houses, management and burials of the extremely infectious dead bodies, psychosocial support and first and foremost solid communication and awareness raising activities with the people in the affected areas are as important as ensuring treatment. Without all of these the disease will continue its spread unhindered. Furthermore, it is of vital importance to ensure a common approach and harmonized methodologies and messages across the region. Therefore a strong

regional coordination is necessary.

6. Case management

An ERU supported by the IFRC and Spanish Red Cross was deployed at the request of the Sierra Leone government in support of Kenema general Hospital. IFRC has shifted its attention to the design and construction of the Ebola Treatment Centre in Kenema. The 60 bed ETC is located 17 kms west of Kenema city. The ETC has 124 local staff employed in a variety of tasks and is supported by an international team of 12. The constraints of limited international staff and the need to train and supervise 164 new local staff has meant that a controlled and steady increase in bed numbers has been planned in phases to ensure staff health and safety. The third and final phase of increase in staff numbers will occur mid October and will allow the unit to meet its full capacity.

Contact information:

Sierra Leone: Constant HS Kargbo, Acting Secretary General, Phone:+233 766 266 74; email: ckargbo@sierraleoneredcross.org

IFRC Sierra Leone: Steve McAndrew, Head of Emergency Operations (HEOPs), Mobile 1 (Sierra Leone): + 232 79 23 67 95, Mobile 2 (Roaming): +41 79 708 4579, email: Stephen.mcandrew@ifrc.org

IFRC Ebola Coordination: Birte Hald, Head of Emergency Operations, IFRC Ebola response, phone: +224 620100615 / +41 79 7084588, email: birte.hald@ifrc.org

IFRC Geneva: Cristina Estrada, Operations Quality Assurance Senior Officer; Geneva; phone: +41 22 730 4260; email: cristina.estrada@ifrc.org

IFRC Africa Zone: Sune Bulow, Disaster Management Delegate for Africa; Nairobi; phone: +254 731 990038; email: sune.bulow@ifrc.org

For Resource Mobilization and Pledges:

IFRC Africa Zone: Martine Zoethoutmaar, Resource Mobilization Coordinator for Africa; Addis Ababa; phone: +251 93 003 4013; email: martine.zoethoutmaar@ifrc.org

14
EBOLA VIRUS: PRESIDENT OBAMA'S SPEECH TO THE UNITED NATIONS

Mr. Secretary General, thank you for bringing us together today to address an urgent threat to the people of West Africa, and a potential threat to the world. Dr. Chan; heads of state and government, especially our partners from Africa; ladies and gentlemen: as we gather here today, the people of Liberia, Guinea and Sierra Leone are in crisis. As Secretary-General Ban and Dr. Chan indicated, the Ebola virus is spreading at an alarming speed. Thousands of men, women and children have died. Thousands more are infected. If unchecked, this epidemic could kill hundreds of thousands of people in the coming months.

Ebola is a horrific disease. It's wiping out whole families. And it has turned simple acts of love and comfort – like holding a sick friend's hand, or embracing a dying child – into potentially fatal acts. If ever there were a public health emergency deserving of an urgent, strong and coordinated international response, this is it.

But this is more than a health crisis. This is a growing threat to regional and global security. In Liberia, Guinea and Sierra Leone, public health systems are near collapse. Economic growth is slowing dramatically. If this epidemic is not stopped, this disease could cause a humanitarian catastrophe across the region. In an era when regional crises can quickly become global threats, stopping Ebola is in the interests of the entire world.

The courageous men and women fighting on the front lines of this disease have told us what they need: more beds, more supplies, and more health workers, as fast as possible. Right now, patients are being left to die in the streets because there's nowhere to put them and no one to help them. One health worker in Sierra Leone compared fighting this outbreak to "fighting a forest fire with spray bottles." With our help, they can put out the blaze.

Last week, I visited the Centers for Disease Control and

Prevention, which is mounting the largest international response in its history. I said that the world could count on America to lead – that we will provide the capabilities that only America has, and mobilize the world the way only America can. And I announced that, in addition to our civilian response, the United States would establish a military command in Liberia to support civilian efforts across the region. Today, that command is up and running.

Our Commander is on the ground in Monrovia, and our teams are working as fast as they can to move in personnel, equipment and supplies. We're working with Senegal to stand up an air bridge to get health workers and medical supplies into West Africa faster. We're setting up a field hospital, which will be staffed by personnel from the U.S. Public Health Service, and a training facility, where we're getting ready to train thousands of health workers from around the world. We're distributing supplies and information kits to hundreds of thousands of families, so they can better protect themselves. And together with our partners, we'll quickly build new treatment units across Liberia, Guinea and Sierra Leone, where thousands will be able to receive care.

Meanwhile, in just the past week, more countries and organizations have stepped up their efforts. So has the United Nations. Mr. Secretary General, the new U.N. Mission for Ebola Emergency Response that you announced last week will bring all the U.N.'s resources to bear in fighting the epidemic, and we thank you for your leadership.

This is progress, and it is encouraging. But we need to be honest with ourselves. It's not enough. There's still a significant gap between where we are and where we need to be. We know from experience that the response to an outbreak of this magnitude needs to be both fast and sustained – like a marathon, but run at the pace of a sprint. That's only possible if every nation and every organization does its part. And everyone has to do more.

International organizations have to move even faster, and mobilize partners on the ground as only they can. More nations need to contribute critical assets and capabilities – whether it's air transport, medical evacuation, health care workers, equipment, or treatment. More foundations can tap into their networks of support, to raise funding and awareness. More businesses, especially those with a presence in the region, can quickly provide their own expertise and resources, from access to critical supply chains to telecommunications. And more citizens – of all nations – can educate themselves on this crisis, contribute to relief efforts and call on their leaders to act. Everyone can do something. That's why we're here today.

And even as we meet the urgent threat of Ebola, it's clear that our nations must do more to prevent, detect and respond to future biological threats – before they erupt into full-blown crises. Tomorrow in Washington, I will host 44 nations to advance our global health security. And we will work with any country that shares that commitment.

Stopping Ebola is a priority for the United States. I've said that this is as important a national security priority for my team as anything else that's out there. We'll do our part. We will continue to lead, but this has to be a priority for everybody else. We cannot do this alone. We don't have the capacity to do all of this by ourselves. We don't have enough health workers by ourselves. We can build the infrastructure and the architecture to get help in, but we're going to need others to contribute.

To my fellow leaders from Liberia, Sierra Leone and Guinea, to the people of West Africa, to the heroic health workers who are on the ground as we speak, in some cases, putting themselves at risk -- I want you to know that you are not alone. We're working urgently to get you the help you need. And we will not stop, we will not relent until we halt this epidemic once and for all. So I want to thank all of you for the efforts that are made.

But I hope that I'm communicating a sense of urgency here. Do not stand by, thinking that it's taken care of. If we don't take care of this now we are going to see fallout effects and secondary effects from this that will have ramifications for a long time, above and beyond the lives that will have been lost.

15
AFTER BEATING EBOLA, NURSE NINA PHAM SHARES A HUG WITH THE PRESIDENT

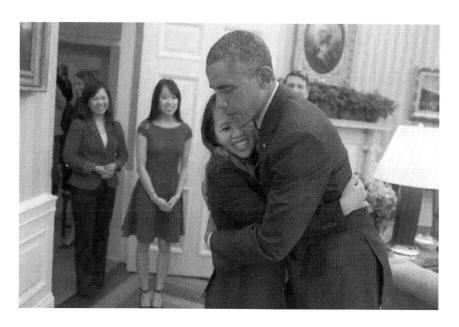

President Barack Obama greets Nina Pham, a Dallas nurse diagnosed with Ebola after caring for an infected patient in Texas, in the Oval Office, Oct. 24, 2014. Pham is virus-free after being treated at the National Institutes of Health Clinical Center in Bethesda, Md. (Official White House Photo by Pete Souza) http://1.usa.gov/1sZudKh

While caring for Ebola patient Thomas Eric Duncan at Texas Health Presbyterian Hospital earlier this month, 26-year-old nurse Nina Pham was also infected with the disease. After first being hospitalized at the Texas hospital, she was later transferred to the National Institutes of Health Clinical Center in Bethesda, Maryland to continue treatment.

But today, 15 days after she first tested positive for Ebola, Nina was declared Ebola-free. Shortly after she left the hospital, President Obama welcomed her to the Oval Office.

At the NIH Clinical Center earlier today, Dr. Anthony Fauci, director of the National Institute of Allergy and Infectious Diseases, announced that Nina was free of the disease, confirming that five separate tests showed she was free of Ebola.

"I feel fortunate and blessed to be standing here today," Nina said in brief remarks to reporters. "I would first and foremost like to thank God, my family, and friends. Throughout this ordeal, I have put my trust in God and my medical team. I am on my way back to recovery, even as I reflect on how many others have not been so fortunate."

The U.S. continues to lead a comprehensive effort to both enhance our preparedness to respond to Ebola here at home, and also combat the epidemic at its source in West Africa. Find out more details on our effort, and get answers to frequently asked questions about Ebola.

**

FACT SHEET: http://1.usa.gov/1pfXN3x
U.S. Response to the Ebola Epidemic in West Africa
As the President has stated, the Ebola epidemic in West Africa and the humanitarian crisis there is a top national security priority for the United States. In order to contain and combat it, we are partnering with the United Nations and other international partners to help the Governments of Guinea, Liberia, Sierra Leone, Nigeria, and Senegal respond just as we fortify our defenses at home. Every outbreak of Ebola over the past 40 years has been contained, and we are confident that this one can—and will be—as well.

Our strategy is predicated on four key goals:
1. Controlling the epidemic at its source in West Africa;
2. Mitigating second-order impacts, including blunting the economic, social, and political tolls in the region;
3. Engaging and coordinating with a broader global audience;
4. Fortifying global health security infrastructure in the region and beyond.

16
WHAT MAKES AMERICA EXCEPTIONAL: PRESIDENT OBAMA THANKS U.S. HEALTH CARE WORKERS FIGHTING EBOLA

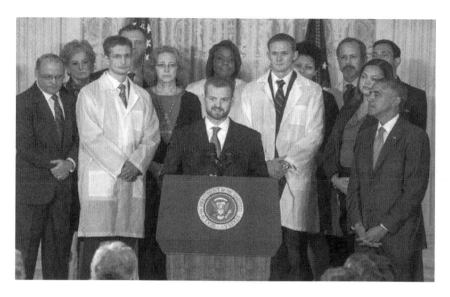

Dr. Kent Brantly delivers remarks during an event with American health care workers fighting Ebola, in the East Room of the White House. October 29, 2014. (Official White House Photo by Chuck Kennedy)

America has never been defined by fear. We are defined by courage and passion and hope and selflessness and sacrifice and a willingness to take on challenges when others can't and others will not, and ordinary Americans who risk their own safety to help those in need, and who inspire, thereby, the example of others -- all in the constant pursuit of building a better world not just for ourselves but for people in every corner of the Earth.

-- President Obama, October 29, 2014 http://1.usa.gov/1s43Gwi

Captain Calvin Edwards is a father of four from Harrisburg, PA. On his 29th wedding anniversary, he left home for Liberia with a pillow and the copy of the New Testament he always carries on his deployments. But not before he bought his wife a dozen roses.

Dr. Dan Chertow is also an officer in the U.S. Public Health Service, who took leave from his position at the National Institutes of Health (NIH) to volunteer with Doctor Without Borders in Liberia, where he cared for more than 200 Ebola patients.

Katie Curren led a "disease detective" team to a village in Sierra Leone that was so remote, they had to take canoes to reach it. The chief who met them wore a Pittsburgh Steelers hat, and welcomed their help. She's completed her mission and is on her way home.

These are just a few of the extraordinary American health workers who are willingly and courageously serving on the frontlines of the Ebola outbreak in West Africa. They signed up to leave their homes and their loved ones to head straight into the heart of the epidemic.

Today in the East Room of the White House, President Obama called on all of us to honor them for what they are: "American heroes" -- a "shining example of what America means to the world, of what is possible when America leads."

When disease or disaster strikes anywhere in the world, the world calls us. And the reason they call us is because of the men and women like the ones who are here today. They respond with skill and professionalism and courage and dedication. And it's because of the determination and skill and dedication and patriotism of folks like this that I'm confident we will contain and ultimately snuff out this outbreak of Ebola -- because that's what we do.

The Ebola outbreak in West Africa is understandably stirring concern at home. But, as the President said, what makes America exceptional is our refusal to hide from the challenges that frighten us most:

We don't react to our fears, but instead, we respond with commonsense and skill and courage. That's the best of our history -- not fear, not hysteria, not misinformation. We react clearly and firmly, even with others are losing their heads. That's part of the reason why we're effective. That's part of the reason why people look to us. And because of the work that's being done by folks like this and by folks who are right now, as we speak, in the three affected countries, we're already seeing a difference.

Our U.S. military and health personnel have been instrumental in setting up supply lines, laying down the necessary transportation infrastructure for aid to get into countries that need it most, cutting the testing time for Ebola by days, doubling safe burial practices, and imbuing a stronger sense of confidence that this outbreak can and will be controlled and defeated.

Still, the problem has not been solved. There is still a severe and significant outbreak, and it will take time for countries to battle back. "We've got a long way to go," the President said. But thanks to American leadership, the mood is changing for the better. "That's what's happening because of American leadership, and it is not abstract: it is people who are willing to go there at significant sacrifice to make a difference. That's American exceptionalism. That's what we should be proud of. That's who we are." Watch his remarks: http://bit.ly/1wV3dkc

We cannot erase the threat of Ebola until we stop the outbreak in West Africa. That is a fact that these health care workers understand, and the mission America is leading on the international stage. The truth is that we are likely to see possible cases outside of the affected countries -- whether or not we adopt a travel ban or a quarantine. That's the nature of diseases. But here's the good news:

We know how to treat this disease. And now that the West African nations of Senegal and Nigeria have been declared Ebola-free, we know that this disease can be contained and defeated if we stay vigilant and committed, and America continues to lead the fight. We've got hundreds of Americans from across the country -- nurses, doctors, public health workers, soldiers, engineers, mechanics -- who are putting themselves on the front lines of this fight. They represent citizenship, and patriotism, and public service at its best. They make huge sacrifices to protect this country that we love. And when they come home, they deserve to be treated properly. They deserve to be treated like the heroes that they are.

The kind of progress that will win the battle against Ebola is slow, it's steady, and it's defined by grace under pressure and courage in the face of fear. It will take the compassion and painstaking effort that these health care providers readily offer. "So I put those on notice who think that we should hide from these problems," the President said. "That's not who we are. That's not who I am. That's not who these folks are. This is America. We do things differently."

That's what I want to see from us -- the pride of a nation that always steps up and gets the job done. America has never been defined by fear. We are defined by courage and passion and hope and selflessness and sacrifice and a willingness to take on challenges when others can't and others will not, and ordinary Americans who risk their own safety to help those in need, and who inspire, thereby, the example of others -- all in the constant pursuit of building a better world not just for ourselves but for people in every corner of the Earth.

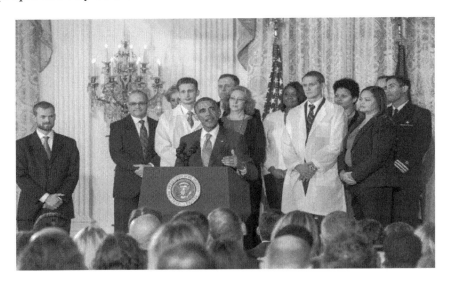

President Barack Obama delivers remarks during an event with American health care workers fighting Ebola, in the East Room of the White House, Oct. 29, 2014. (Official White House Photo by Pete Souza)

17 SOCIAL MEDIA & EBOLA

With news of the first diagnosed case of Ebola in the U.S., the public is on edge and turning to social media for fast answers about just how vulnerable they are to the deadly virus.

For even the most skilled Twitter maven, providing accurate information on Ebola in 140 characters or less is a challenge. Social media is sometimes a challenging place to deal with complex subjects, but it's a way to reach millions of people, so public health officials and medical experts are using Twitter and Facebook to try to educate and inform.

But other users take to the same outlets to share half-truths and rumors, perpetuating a number of irrational fears about Ebola. Misinformation can spread much faster across the U.S. than the virus ever could.

Many Twitter users have tried to combat the gross misunderstandings in circulation, especially about how the virus is contracted and how to recognize symptoms. In an effort to combat the virtual hysteria, many health and government organizations are harnessing social media to educate the public about the realities of the disease.

CDC #DiseaseDetectives answered questions on #Ebola in #CDCchat. Check out our new storify & get the facts http://bit.ly/1vU4qHd http://t.co/5a7cTu2vly

CBS Evening News @CBSEveningNews · Oct 8
Using Twitter to inoculate the public against ignorance about Ebola: cbsn.ws/1y8Zy57

NewsHour @NewsHour · Oct 9
Meet the disease detectives tracking #Ebola at the #CDC to.pbs.org/1vOXLib

**

ABOUT THE AUTHOR

Thomas Baker is the Past-President of TESOL Chile. He is also the Co-Founder and Co-Organiser of EdCamp Santiago, which provides free, participant-driven professional development for teachers, by teachers.

Thomas is a writer, teacher, and teacher-trainer who has lived in Chile for the past fifteen years. The source and inspiration for his writing comes from his family.

My blog can be found at http://www.profesorbaker.com.

Other books by Thomas: http://amzn.to/1A6tj56 .

Made in the USA
Lexington, KY
12 April 2015